BRADY

Emergency Responder

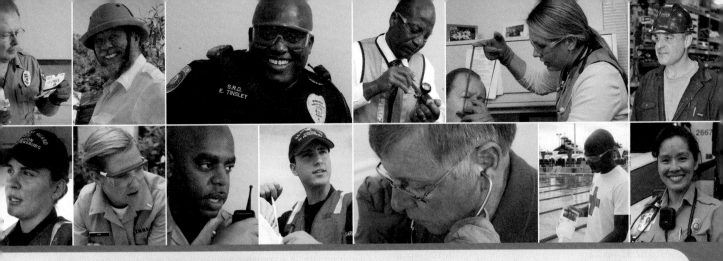

IIBRADY

Emergency Responder

Advanced First Aid for Non-EMS Personnel

Christopher J. Le Baudour

Medical Editor
Keith Wesley, MD

Brady
is an imprint of

Pearson

Boston   Columbus   Indianapolis   New York   San Francisco   Upper Saddle River
Amsterdam   Cape Town   Dubai   London   Madrid   Milan   Munich   Paris
Montreal   Toronto   Delhi   Mexico City   Sao Paulo   Sydney   Hong Kong
Seoul   Singapore   Taipei   Tokyo

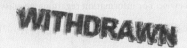

Library of Congress Cataloging-in-Publication Data

Le Baudour, Chris.
   Emergency responder : advanced first aid for non-EMS personnel /
Christopher J. Le Baudour ; medical reviewer, Keith Wesley.
      p. ; cm.
   Includes bibliographical references and index.
   ISBN-13: 978-0-13-171214-0
   ISBN-10: 0-13-171214-4
   1. First aid in illness and injury.   2. Medical emergencies.
   I. Wesley, Keith.   II. Title.
   [DNLM: 1. First Aid—methods.   2. Rescue Work.
   3. Emergencies.   4. Moving and Lifting Patients.   5. Needs
   Assessment.   6. Wounds and Injuries. WA 292]

   RC86.7.L4 2012
   616.02'52—dc22   2010034066

Publisher: Julie Levin Alexander
Publisher's Assistant: Regina Bruno
Editor-in-Chief: Marlene McHugh Pratt
Acquisitions Editor: Sladjana Repic
Senior Managing Editor for Development: Lois Berlowitz
Project Manager: Josephine Cepeda
Editorial Assistant: Jonathan Cheung
Director of Marketing: David Gesell
Executive Marketing Manager: Katrin Beacom
Marketing Manager: Brian Hoehl
Marketing Specialist: Michael Sirinides
Managing Editor for Production: Patrick Walsh
Production Liaison: Faye Gemmellaro
Production Editor: Peggy Kellar, Aptara®, Inc.
Manufacturing Manager: Ilene Sanford
Manufacturing Buyer: Alan Fischer
Art Director: Kristine Carney
Cover and Interior Design: Laura Ierardi, LCI Design
Managing Photography Editor: Michal Heron
Photographer: Michal Heron
Editorial Media Manager: Amy Peltier
Media Project Manager: Lorena Cerisano
Composition: Aptara®, Inc.
Printer/Binder: RR Donnelley
Cover Printer: Lehigh-Phoenix Color/Hagerstown

Many of the designations by manufacturers and sellers to distinguish their products are claimed as trademarks. Where those designations appear in this book, and the publisher was aware of a trademark claim, the designations have been printed in initial caps or all caps.

Notice: The author and the publisher of this book have taken care to make certain that the information given is correct and compatible with the standards generally accepted at the time of publication. Nevertheless, as new information becomes available, changes in treatment and in the use of equipment and procedures become necessary. The reader is advised to carefully consult the instruction and information material included in each piece of equipment or device before administration. Students are warned that the use of any techniques must be authorized by their medical advisor, where appropriate, in accordance with local laws and regulations. The publisher disclaims any liability, loss, injury, or damage incurred as a consequence, directly or indirectly, of the use and application of any of the contents of this book.

Notice on Gender Usage: The English language has historically given preference to the male gender. Among many words, the pronouns *he* and *his* are commonly used to describe both genders. Society evolves faster than language, and the male pronouns still predominate in our speech. The author has made great effort to treat the two genders equally, recognizing that a significant percentage of responders and patients are female. However, in some instances, male pronouns may be used to describe both male and female responders and patients solely for the purpose of brevity. This is not intended to offend any readers of the female gender.

Brady
is an imprint of

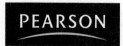

www.bradybooks.com

10 9 8 7 6 5 4 3 2 1
ISBN 13: 978-0-13-171214-0
ISBN 10:   0-13-171214-4

DEDICATION

This textbook and the entire program that it represents are dedicated to the army of individuals across this country who represent non-EMS personnel and who demonstrate immense courage by stepping out of their comfort zone and volunteer to serve the needs of others in their time of need.

"One thing I know: the only ones among you who will be really happy are those who will have sought and found how to serve."

—Dr. Albert Schweitzer

Contents

CHAPTER 10   **Caring for Muscle and Bone Injuries**   135

CHAPTER 11   **Caring for Injuries to the Head and Spine**   150

Photo Scans

Letter to Students

On behalf of the entire team of dedicated individuals who helped make this important resource available to you, I'd like to welcome you to *Emergency Responder: Advanced First Aid for Non-EMS Personnel*. My name is Chris Le Baudour, and I am both proud and humbled to count myself among the hundreds of thousands of individuals like you who have learned the skills necessary to assist those who become ill or injured unexpectedly.

I believe that we have assembled an innovative educational program unlike any other—a program designed specifically to meet the needs of those of you who have accepted the additional responsibility of caring for the ill and injured during an emergency. You are a unique group of professionals whose primary job might be serving as a law enforcement officer, firefighter, life guard, correctional officer, emergency response team member, security officer, or any one of a dozen other vocations not directly related to providing emergency first aid. You are unique because you have decided and in most cases volunteered to receive additional training so that you will be better prepared to provide lifesaving first-aid care to someone stricken with a sudden illness or injury.

One of the questions we struggled with when developing this program was what to call you, the individuals who would be receiving this training. You fill a unique void between the person with basic first-aid training and the person with the first level of EMS training, referred to as the Emergency Medical Responder (formerly First Responder). The term *first responder* as we use it in this textbook refers to any individual who may happen upon the scene of an emergency regardless if he or she has received training. You, of course, fall into this category, but because of the more advanced training that you will be receiving, we also will be referring to you as Emergency Responders. As Emergency Responders you are a very important first link in the chain of care that begins with you and continues with the EMS system and finally the care provided at the hospital.

This educational program is designed for the working professionals who must attend to their normal job duties and still find time to participate in this training program. It is a flexible program that blends this textbook with instructor-led hands-on training events. Depending on the needs of the organization and the students, this modular program can be delivered in as few as 15 hours and may extend up to 24 hours.

We want to emphasize that all emergency training should include adequate time for hands-on skills training. It is not enough simply to read about how to care for the ill and injured; you must practice the basic skills that will be required to perform your duties well. We have carefully selected those skills that we believe will be the most important for you to learn in order to care for the most life-threatening events. We also have included carefully designed skill sheets that will assist you in developing the competency necessary to perform each skill with accuracy and confidence.

We would like to encourage you to continue on beyond your initial training once you complete this course. You always can refer to this textbook or review the online modules. Doing so will help keep your knowledge and skills sharp and ready for when they are needed. We are pleased that you have decided to participate in this valuable training program and applaud you for your dedication to the service of others in their time of most need. If you ever have a desire to contact us for any reason, you may do so by e-mailing me at chris@icarevalues.org.

We look forward to your comments and suggestions!

Respectfully,
Chris Le Baudour

Preface

EMERGENCY RESPONDER TRAINING PROGRAM

Planning and development for this book have been in the works for nearly five years, and we are proud to see that it is finally in your hands. The world of emergency response has undergone many changes over the past several years and is still doing so. I personally have spent the better part of the past 20 years training and developing Emergency Response Teams within a wide variety of environments, from corporations to industry to municipalities and school districts. Over the past several years, we have seen a steady increase in the desire of these teams to learn more about how best to care for those that become ill or injured while on the job. This book is just one piece of the overall program to help address this growing need.

ABOUT THIS TEXTBOOK

Comprehensive Learning Program

This is not just another first-aid book. This textbook represents many years of experience teaching and training in the pre-EMS environment and is just one element in a comprehensive program designed to meet the needs of you the student, the instructor, and your employer. We have provided instructors with an instructor's resource CD, which contains tools to customize a training program specifically for your environment. And we have provided students with online course material as an adjunct to textbook learning.

Great care was taken in designing the learning path for this program. We begin with many of the foundational principles necessary to understand the scope of your new role as well as the information to keep you safe and healthy along the way. We carefully build on that foundation and add knowledge and the appropriate skills in a very logical and meaningful manner.

DEPTH AND BREADTH OF CONTENT

The textbook contains 13 chapters and four appendices. It starts by introducing you to the basic concepts of emergency medical care, EMS, and how you will be expected to perform in your role as an Emergency Responder. We then present in a logical and easy-to-follow format many of the most common illnesses and injuries you are likely to encounter. We provide a realistic depth and breadth of information and in a way that we know will make you successful with caring for the people who have fallen victim to sudden illness or injury. The material in the appendices is slightly more advanced and may be optional, depending on the responsibilities you will have in your jurisdiction.

FEATURES

Each chapter in *Emergency Responder* begins with the same four elements: (1) comprehensive learning objectives that provide the solid foundation for what you will be expected to learn and perform; (2) a list of key terms that will introduce you to the new vocabulary essential to your overall understanding of the content; (3) an introduction that sets the stage for the instructional narrative that follows; and (4) "The Emergency," a scenario that places you at the scene of a realistic emergency and asks you to think about what you might feel, think, say, and do as you read the text and apply your newfound knowledge.

At the conclusion of each chapter you will find "The Handoff," which brings closure to the opening scenario, "The Emergency," in a way that applies all you have learned in the chapter. Following "The Handoff" is the chapter review, which includes the chapter summary, a concise review of the chapter's key points, and a Quick Quiz, which offers multiple-choice questions that help you test how well you understand the key concepts and information covered in the chapter.

Look for helpful study aids within the chapter as well. One such study aid is the Quick Check, which intersperses open-ended questions throughout the instructional narrative. The Quick Check will help you stop, think, and apply the information you've just read. In the margins, you'll find your learning objectives, positioned right beside the corresponding sections of the chapter, and you'll find the key terms and definitions placed where each one is first introduced and discussed.

We are pleased that you have chosen to serve in this manner and know that this learning program will be a valuable resource for your initial training and as a reference tool for many years to come.

Welcome aboard!

Introduction to American Safety and Health Institute (ASHI)

This book is an important element of the complete training and certification program offered by qualified instructors affiliated with the training centers approved by the American Safety and Health Institute (ASHI). The EMS system of care begins with those who are first to recognize that an emergency exists and apply accepted principles of life-supporting care and appropriate first aid. An Emergency Responder is a formally trained individual who arrives first on the scene of an incident and takes action to save lives. The ASHI Emergency Responder training program is designed to fill the knowledge and skill gap between basic first-aid training and EMS. Non-EMS personnel who will benefit from this training program include public and private safety, security, and service personnel, including firefighters, law enforcement officers, park rangers, customs agents, lifeguards, correctional officers, members of business emergency response teams, camp health officers, counselors, coaches, and other interested persons requiring (or desiring) advanced first-aid certification.

ASHI Emergency Responder Certification Card

Evaluation of knowledge and skill competence is required for ASHI certification as an Emergency Responder. The learner must successfully complete the ASHI Emergency Responder exam and demonstrate the ability to work as an Emergency Responder in a scenario-based team setting, adequately directing the primary assessment and care of responsive and unresponsive medical and trauma patients.

AMERICAN ■SAFETY& HEALTH■ INSTITUTE

A member of the
HSI family of brands

THE AMERICAN SAFETY AND HEALTH INSTITUTE

The American Safety and Health Institute (ASHI) is a leading provider of emergency care training programs for qualified instructors. With a customer base of roughly 35,000 professional educators and more than 5,500 training centers around the world, ASHI trains instructors from a variety of backgrounds. Many are current or former Emergency Medical Technicians, firefighters, and other Emergency Responders who consider emergency care training both a passion and a profession.

Regulatory Compliance

Laws, regulations, and organizational approval policies frequently change, and unless otherwise provided, ASHI makes no representations or warranties as to whether a given program meets specific occupational licensing, certification, or policy requirements for a specific state agency or other approval authority. *Emergency Responder* does not include training or certification in cardiopulmonary resuscitation and should not be used for that purpose.

Certification

In support of a systems approach to emergency medical care, content for ASHI Emergency Responder training is based on National Emergency Medical Services (EMS) Education Standards. Certification does imply EMS state licensure or credentialing and is not a guarantee of future performance.

American Safety and Health Institute
1450 Westec Drive, Eugene, OR 97402
Phone 800–800-7099, Fax 541–344-7429

Acknowledgments

I constantly remind my students that responding to the needs of others during an emergency is a team sport. It takes the efforts of many to render first aid efficiently and appropriately every time. Assembling a project such as this is no exception. Without the coordinated efforts of many people spread throughout the United States, this project could not have been possible. I'd like to use this space to acknowledge the key players who helped identify the need, form the vision, and create the end product that you see before you.

I'd like to begin with Ralph Shenefelt, Vice President of Regulatory and QA at the American Safety and Health Institute (ASHI), for his clear vision and ability to see a need. Although I have spent many years helping develop and train non-EMS personnel, Ralph helped identify the need for a project with the exact depth and breadth to address this underserved provider. I'd like to express my appreciation for Mr. Bill Rowe, of the Health and Safety Institute (HSI), for his wisdom, guidance, and dedication to quality education for the pre-EMS provider.

Thanks to Audrey Le Baudour, my personal assistant, copy editor, travel coordinator, and last but not least, my wife, the one who keeps me organized, focused, and, most importantly, on schedule.

I'd like to say thank you to Lieutenant Brad Dykens of St. Petersburg Fire and Rescue for all his time and effort assisting with the coordination and logistics of the photo shoot in Florida.

I'd like to extend a special thank you to our photographer, Michal Heron, who has singlehandedly raised the bar for the way EMS is depicted in textbooks across this country. Michal, you bring something that no other artist brings when shooting for these books. Your work is clearly head and shoulders above the rest, and you really challenge authors to do it better.

I'd like to say thank you to Editor in Chief Marlene Pratt, Acquisitions Editor Sladjana Repic, Senior Managing Editor for Development Lois Berlowitz, and Development Editor Jo Cepeda for their invaluable editorial assistance and eye on quality. I'd also like to extend my appreciation to Jonathan Cheung and Monica Moosang and the entire sales team at Pearson Education, who provide the support and infrastructure to make these projects happen and get to those who need them. The skill and teamwork it takes to choreograph a project such as this is truly amazing.

MEDICAL EDITOR

Keith Wesley, MD, FACEP

Dr. Wesley is the Wisconsin State EMS Medical Director and is a board-certified emergency medicine physician living in Eau Claire, Wisconsin. He is the chair of the National Council of State EMS Medical Directors. Dr. Wesley is the author of many articles and EMS textbooks and is a frequent speaker at EMS conferences across the nation. He is an active EMS medical director currently providing medical oversight to the Chippewa Fire District in Chippewa Falls, Wisconsin; to EMT-Basic Services of Ashland and Bayfield counties; and to the Apostle Islands Lake Shore National Park.

CONTRIBUTORS

We would like to express special appreciation to the following specialist who contributed to chapter development:

Brian D. Bricker, EMT, CFC
  REACH Air Medical, Santa Rosa, CA

REVIEWERS

We would like to thank the following reviewers for providing invaluable feedback, insight, and suggestions in preparation of *Emergency Responder: Advanced First Aid for Non-EMS Personnel:*

John L. Beckman, FF/EMT-P, AA, BS
  Fire Science Instructor, Technology Center of DuPage/Addison Fire Protection District, Addison, IL
Raymond W. Burton, Deputy Major
  Plymouth County Sheriff's Department; Instructor-Trainer, Plymouth Regional Police Academy, Plymouth, MA
Kim Dennison, RN, BSN, COHC
  Owner of Absolute Learning Success, LLC.; occupational health and safety nurse, Perry, MI
Andy Dunford, EMT-I
  Operations Manager, Stone Ambulance Service, Inc., Martinsville, VA
Jeanne Hanson, BSc, EMT-B
  President, Mountain Medic CPR, Snohomish County, WA
Richard Huff
  Chief, Atlantic Highlands First Aid and Safety Squad, Atlantic Highlands, NJ
Kenneth M. Knight, NREMT-P
  Bakersfield, CA
R. Scott Lauder, RN
  Chief Executive Officer, Initial Response, Inc., Smithfield, VA
Alan P. McCartney, CSP, CFPS, RPIH, EMT-P
  Safety Officer/Paramedic, Bradford Fire and Rescue, Bradford, NH
Deborah L. Petty, BS, CICP, EMT-P I/C
  Paramedic Training Officer, Training Academy, St. Charles County Ambulance District, St. Peters, MO
Steve Thomas, EMT-P
  Director of Training, Alert CPR Emergency Training, Lewisville, TX
Carl Voskamp, MBA, Lic.P.
  EMS Program Coordinator, The Victoria College, Victoria, TX

Steve Yarberry
Regional Coordinator, Forrest City, AR
Jerry Young-Kilmer, M.Ed.
Curriculum Development Specialist, Washington Department of Corrections, Spokane, WA

PHOTO ACKNOWLEDGMENTS

All photographs not credited adjacent to the photograph or in a photo credit section were photographed on assignment for Brady Prentice Hall Pearson Education.

ORGANIZATIONS

We wish to thank the following organizations for their assistance in creating the new photo program:

American Safety and Health Institute
Mary Ann Herbel, Logistics Coordinator

American Safety and Health Institute
William Rowe, Firefighter/Paramedic (ret.); Director, Product Development

American Safety and Health Institute
Ralph M. Shenefelt, Firefighter/Paramedic (ret.); Vice President of Regulatory and QA

St. Petersburg (FL) Fire and Rescue
Bradford A. Dykens, Lieutenant, EMTP

St. Petersburg (FL) College
Lauren Dupont, Coordinator, CJ Academies Department

Southeastern Public Safety Institute
John Dressback, Program Director, Southeastern Public Safety Institute, St. Petersburg (FL) College

City of St. Petersburg (FL) Recreation Department, North Shore Pool
Mario L. Abadal, Recreation Supervisor

United States Coast Guard Station, St. Petersburg (FL)
BMCS Sean Benton

University of South Florida Campus Police
Chief Rene Chenevert

PHOTO ASSISTANT AND COMPUTER POSTPRODUCTION

Ken Lopez, *Orlando, FL*
Doug Cupid, *Orlando, FL*

TECHNICAL ADVISORS

Thanks to the following people for providing technical support during the new photo shoots:

Bradford A. Dykens, Lieutenant, EMTP
> *St. Petersburg (FL) Fire and Rescue*

Fredrick H. (Ted) Rogers, BA, NREMT-P
> *Lead EMT Instructor, St. Petersburg (FL) College EMS Program*

Thank you to the following for supplying locations for the new photo shoots:

Tino Mastry, President
> *Mastry Engine Center, 2801 Anvil Street North, St. Petersburg, FL*

CDR Robert Gibbons
> *Admiral Farragut Academy, 501 Park Street North, St. Petersburg, FL*

Location Logistical Assistance
Debra Dykens, *Admiral Farragut Academy*

PHOTOGRAPHY MODELS

Thanks to the following people from the St. Petersburg (FL) area who portrayed patients and EMS providers in the new photographs:

Devora Ballo
William T. Ballo
Luciana Belfiglio
Andrew M. Bittner
Sara Brown
Christian Cain
Brittany Caruso
Kate Cillian
Anthony Cooley
Patricia Delfin
Kevin DeLoatch
Robert DeMario
Lauren DuPont
Jonathan Dye
Bradford Dykens
Dana M. Dykens
Shelby Erb
Gerald Gladstone

Michael Goodnight
Kathy Henderson
Mitch Heykoop
Kermit Michel Hunter II
Mitch Incorvaia
Norma P. Jackson
James M. Quinlon
Fredrick H. Rogers
Ralph Shenefelt
Craig Smith
Joseph Smith
Chris Tidwell
Eric D. Tinsley
Hermann Trappman
Ritsuki Umeda
Carol A. Vassillion
K. Louise Williams

United States Coast Guard Station, St. Petersburg, FL:

Jennifer Catlin
Keith Crumpe
Nathan Jones

Juan Lebron
Michael Meadows
Jason White

About the Author

Christopher J. Le Baudour

Christopher Le Baudour has been working in Emergency Medical Services (EMS) since 1978 in both field and clinical settings. In 1984, he began his teaching career in the Department of Public Safety, EMS Division, at Santa Rosa Junior College in Santa Rosa, California.

Chris holds a Master's Degree in Education with an emphasis in online teaching and learning, as well as numerous certifications. He has spent the past 25 years mastering the art of experiential learning in EMS and is well known for his innovative classroom techniques and his passion for teaching and learning in both traditional and online classrooms.

Chris is very involved in EMS education at the national level, serving as a board member of the National Association of EMS Educators, as well as being active on many subcommittees. He has been a keynote speaker at both state and national conferences and is a prolific EMS writer. Chris and Audrey, his wife of 24 years, have two children and reside in northern California.

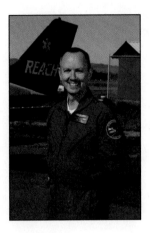

Emergency Responder:
ADVANCED FIRST AID FOR NON-EMS PERSONNEL

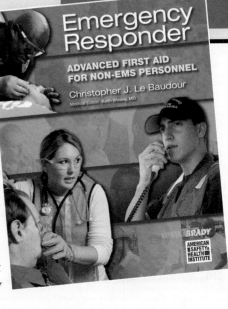

Dear Instructor:

Brady, your destination for education, is pleased to bring you the first edition of *Emergency Responder: Advanced First Aid for Non-EMS Personnel.* This new solution is an important component of a complete training program for responders who are trained to provide first aid before EMS personnel arrive. Regardless of the responder's primary occupation—law enforcement officer, firefighter, life guard, corrections officer, corporate response team member, security officer, park ranger, or other—this program is designed to provide users with the knowledge and skills necessary to take them beyond basic first-aid training so they can provide better care. This manual presents in a logical and easy-to-follow format many of the most common illnesses and injuries that Emergency Responders are likely to encounter in their professions.

For many years now, Brady, the leading publisher in EMS, has partnered with the American Safety and Health Institute (ASHI), a nationally recognized provider of emergency care training programs for authorized instructors and approved training centers to provide complete and comprehensive training and certification programs. This new training and certification solution builds on our past success and is designed to help fill the knowledge and skill gap that exists between very basic first aid training and certification and the extensive training and certification required for EMS professionals. Though designed as a complete certification program, this text can be used for training without ASHI certification.

The following walkthrough outlines the features found throughout the manual. It also provides information about instructor resources that can be used to make your program experience the best it can be.

We thank you for choosing *Emergency Responder: Advanced First Aid for Non-EMS Personnel.* We are proud to continue our tradition of bringing the highest standards of authorship, content development, production, support, and service that our customers expect and deserve.

Sincerely,

Marlene McHugh Pratt
Editor-in-Chief

Lois Berlowitz
Senior Managing Editor

Thomas Kennally
Director of Sales

Sladjana Repic
Acquisitions Editor

Brian Hoehl
Marketing Manager

Guide to Key Features

◀ **Learning Objectives** Each chapter begins with a list of the objectives that forms the basis of material. The page on which each objective is covered is also included. Within the chapter, marginal references appear as close as possible to the specific objectives being addressed.

◀ **Key Terms** These appear at the beginning of each chapter, in addition to the page number on which the term is first presented. Also, each term is defined in text margins.

MAKE A NOTE

Mental status is not something you just assess once at the beginning of an assessment. It is a continuous process that occurs throughout your time with the person. Pay close attention to how the person responds to your questions and to the environment around him. Changes in responses may indicate that the person is getting worse or better. ●

▲ **Make a Note** Highlights important, need-to-know information.

The Emergency ▶ Scenarios challenge the student to consider his or her role and responsibilities and determine patient care priorities. These appear at the start of each chapter.

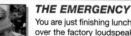

THE EMERGENCY

You are just finishing lunch when you hear a piercing tone over the factory loudspeakers followed by the operator's echoing voice. "Attention all Emergency Response Team members. Please respond to the level-two mezzanine." You have been on the company's Emergency Response Team for two months, and this is the first time that you have been summoned. Your heart begins racing and your hands shake slightly as you throw your sandwich wrapper and napkin into the garbage can on your way out of the lunchroom.

The level-two mezzanine, a plain concrete walkway overlooking the bustling production lines below, appears empty from your vantage point as the cargo elevator rumbles up to the main level. As the cage doors scrape open, you grab the red ERT bag from its place on the shelf and rush to the skeletal staircase leading to the mezzanine.

Reaching the top of the stairs, you see that Frank, the dayshift production supervisor, is lying on his back on the mezzanine.

"Thank heavens you're here!" Frank's assistant, Trina, runs up from the opposite end of the walkway. "We were talking and he just kind of slumped into the wall and passed out. I helped him to the floor and ran and called for help."

"Well, the scene is safe," you say to yourself, looking around the mezzanine and factory below. "It doesn't seem to be a trauma. Did he hit his head or twist his neck when you helped him to the ground?"

"No." Trina shakes her head vigorously. "I was really gentle."

You kneel next to Frank and immediately notice how pale his face is. "Frank!" you shout, gently shaking his shoulder. "Frank, I need you to wake up!"

There is no response, and as you lean down to check on Frank's breathing you instruct Trina to go get the defibrillator and make sure that the operator has contacted 911 to activate local EMS.

QUICK CHECK

What is the term used to describe the general nature of a person's injury? Of a person's illness? ●

▲ **Quick Check** Questions that test knowledge of key content in the manual.

SAFETY CHECK

You are not obligated to help an ill or injured person if it puts you at risk. You must first do your best to ensure that all immediate risks have been mitigated before entering the scene. If you cannot mitigate a risk, do not enter the scene. Call 911 and wait for the appropriate resources to take over. ●

◀ **Safety Check** Emphasizes specific safety considerations for the Emergency Responder.

PEDIATRIC CARE

Beginning your assessment at the head can be very frightening for a child. In an effort to build trust, begin your assessment at the child's feet and work your way up to the head. Of course, if there are issues related to the ABCs (airway, breathing, circulation), you always would begin at the head. ●

▲ **Pediatric Care** Highlights unique experiences and considerations when dealing with this special population.

The Handoff This is the conclusion of The Emergency scenario that appears at the beginning of the chapter.

▼

Skill Scans ▶
Step-by-step visual layouts on how to perform skills.

SCAN 7.4   **Locating the Radial Pulse Point**

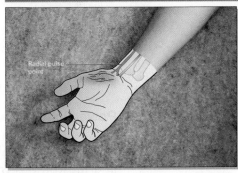

7.4.1 Locating the radial pulse point.

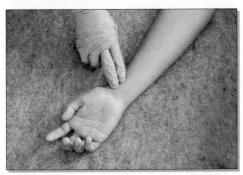

7.4.2 Feeling for the presence of a radial pulse.

THE HANDOFF

You are on your third cycle of chest compressions on Frank when Trina scrambles back up to the mezzanine with the AED hanging over her shoulder, banging against her hip.

"The fire department is just coming up the elevator with the other ERT members," she says breathlessly. "They should all be here in a minute."

You continue chest compressions as Trina opens the AED, turns it on, and with shaking hands places the foam electrodes on the man.

"You're doing great," you say to her, taking deep breaths and sweating as the AED analyzes Frank's heart rhythm. "You put those pads on perfectly."

You hear a multitude of feet clumping up the stairs behind you as the AED voice says, "Shock advised." After it charges, you make sure that neither you nor Trina is touching Frank before pushing the large blinking button.

"What happened?" A firefighter squats next to you as the AED is analyzing Frank again.

"Uh, he was apparently just walking with Trina and passed out." You wipe sweat from your forehead with a gloved hand. "And when I got here he wasn't breathing and had no signs of life, so I started CPR and it shocked him once just now, and—"

"Resume CPR," the machine's [...]

"We've got it." Two of the firefi[...] move out of their way.

Soon the AED demands a seco[...] moves his arm and begins to breath[...]

"That's amazing," Rhoann, a fe[...] whispers loudly into your ear as sh[...] job assessing the situation and Fra[...]

Chapter Summary ▶
End-of-chapter summary gives a concise review of important chapter information.

CHAPTER REVIEW

Chapter Summary

● All ill or injured persons can be categorized based on the mechanism of injury or nature of illness.

● Signs and symptoms are indicators that you will look for and evaluate as part of your assessment. A sign is something you can see, while a symptom is something the person tells you about the situation.

● The components of an assessment include the scene size-up, primary assessment, secondary assessment, and th[...] is mostly about [...] assessment is a[...] threats. The se[...]

physical examination and history. The reassessment includes reevaluating the assessment and any required interventions.

● Mental status can be assessed using the AVPU scale (alert, verbal, painful, unresponsive).

● The SAMPLE history tool stands for signs and symptoms, allergies, medications, past medical history, last oral intake, and events leading up to

Quick Quiz At the end of ▶ every chapter, multiple-choice review questions directly tied to the learning objectives are provided.

Quick Quiz

1. All of the following are examples of symptoms EXCEPT:
   a. nausea.
   b. cool skin.
   c. pain.
   d. fatigue.

2. Which one of the following describes the nature of illness?
   a. The person fell from a roof.
   b. The person has a badly twisted ankle.
   c. The person was struck in the head.
   d. The person is experiencing difficulty breathing.

3. Specific care that you provide to an ill or injured person is called a(n):

7. The O in the BP-DOC mnemonic stands for:
   a. open wounds.
   b. oral history.
   c. observable injuries.
   d. occlusions.

8. You are approached by a coworker who was injured during her lunch break. She tells you that her left wrist hurts and denies pain elsewhere. You should initially try to determine:
   a. the nature of her illness.
   b. what her medical history is.
   c. her chief complaint.
   d. the mechanism of injury.

9. You are at a family event and one of your relatives [...]

Teaching Package

The following instructor resources are available to help you achieve success in the classroom.

Instructor's Resource Manual (ISBN 0-13-224156-0)
This guide includes objectives, presentation outlines, handouts with answer keys, quizzes, and unique classroom activities designed to engage students.

PowerPoint™ Presentation with Instructor Notes (ISBN 0-13-230169-5)
This resource includes more than 500 customizable slides that make your lectures truly visual. Slides present key concepts with impactful photographs and illustrations from the text. Instructor's notes reinforce content on the slides and provide a script for presentation.

MyTest Program (ISBN 0-13-238039-0)
This program contains multiple-choice questions that support and reinforce textbook manual content. MyTest software can be used to customize your tests and present questions electronically or on paper. You can also add your own questions to the database. Answer keys, text page references, and objective references are also provided.

For more information on these resources and how to access them from our Instructor's Resource Center, please contact your Brady sales representative.

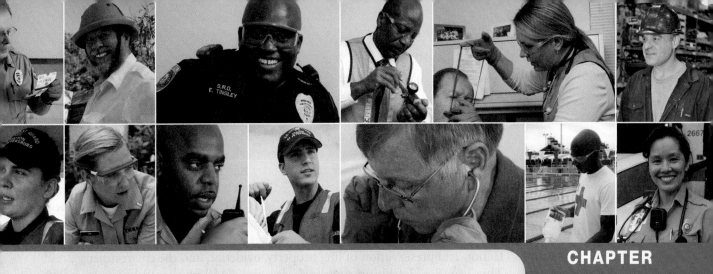

Introduction to EMS Systems and the Role of the Emergency Responder

LEARNING OBJECTIVES

At the conclusion of this chapter and the associated instructor-guided lesson, the student will be able to:

Cognitive

1.1 Identify the common components of an emergency medical services (EMS) system. *(p. 3)*

1.2 Differentiate among the four levels of EMS providers. *(p. 4)*

1.3 Differentiate among the roles and responsibilities of the Emergency Responder from other EMS providers. *(p. 6)*

1.4 Explain the role that the Emergency Responder plays in ensuring the safety of all people at the scene of an emergency. *(p. 6)*

1.5 Explain the various methods used to access the EMS system. *(p. 8)*

1.6 Explain the concept of medical direction and how it relates to the Emergency Responder. *(p. 8)*

KEY TERMS

The following terms are introduced in this chapter:

- emergency medical services (EMS) *(p. 3)*
- Emergency Responder *(p. 2)*
- medical direction *(p. 8)*
- Medical Director *(p. 8)*
- protocols *(p. 8)*

Introduction

EACH year in the United States there are over 4 million workplace illnesses and injuries.[1] A sudden illness or injury can happen at any time without warning—at home, at work, or while on vacation. No one wants to think about that, but everyone knows the possibility exists. As an Emergency Responder, you become part of the system to aid those stricken by a sudden illness or injury.

The term *first responder* traditionally has been used to describe the first level of training and certification for emergency medical service (EMS) personnel, but since the events of September 11, 2001, the definition has broadened. Homeland Security Presidential Directive 8 defines *first responders* as "those individuals who in the early stages of an incident are responsible for the protection and preservation of life, property, evidence, and the environment. . . ."[2] This broader definition now includes non-EMS public and private safety, security, and service personnel, including firefighters, law enforcement officers, lifeguards, correctional officers, security officers, members of business and corporate emergency response teams, and members of emergency management, public health, and corporate and industrial response teams, among others. Simply put, an **Emergency Responder** is any individual with formal training who arrives first on the scene of an incident and takes action to protect bystanders and save lives (▼ Figure 1.1).

Emergency Responder an individual who arrives first on the scene of an incident and takes action to protect bystanders and to save lives.

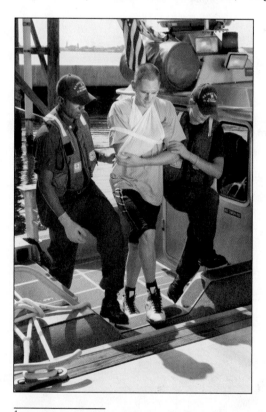

Figure 1.1 As an Emergency Responder, you will provide care for ill and injured persons until EMS arrives.

---

[1]Occupational Safety and Health Administration, *Best Practices Guide: Fundamentals of a Workplace First-Aid Program*. OSHA 3317–06N 2006 (Washington, DC: U.S. Department of Labor, 2006), 4. Also available online at http://www.osha.gov/Publications/OSHA3317first-aid.pdf (accessed January 10, 2010).

[2]U.S. Department of Homeland Security, *Homeland Security Directive 8: National Preparedness* (Washington, DC: U.S. Department of Homeland Security, 2003), http://www.dhs.gov/xabout/laws/gc_1215444247124.shtm (accessed January 10, 2010).

This book is an important element of a complete training program for responders who are trained to provide first-aid care before EMS personnel arrive. Regardless of your primary occupation, it is designed to provide you with the knowledge and skills necessary to take you beyond basic first-aid training and help you learn to provide emergency medical care for the most common medical emergencies.

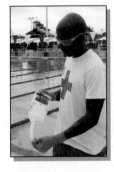

THE EMERGENCY

The cool scent of chlorinated water mingled with sunscreen rises to your perch on the lifeguard chair as you spend another summer afternoon listening to laughter, screams, and thunderous splashes at your city's only public pool. You continuously scan the area, left to right, far to near. The occasional shrill note from the whistle kept clamped in your teeth warns the girls to stop running along the concrete or the boys from getting too rough with friends in the deep end. You note the position of the sun and twist the base of the large white umbrella so that the cool shade covers you.

"Help!" A woman's scream cuts through the noise of the crowded pool area. "Somebody help him!"

You immediately stand up on the top rung of the chair ladder and scan the dripping crowd for the source of the yelling. At the far end of the pool, you see a teenage boy lying on the wet concrete with a woman kneeling next to him, the brim of her large hat bobbing as she yells at him to wake up.

"Everyone out of the water!" you shout, your voice amplified by a bull-horn mounted to the platform. Satisfied that the swimmers are moving out of the pool in an orderly fashion, you drop the microphone and scramble down the ladder. You grab the orange response bag from the shelf at the base of the lifeguard tower and then walk quickly to where a group is beginning to gather.

"He slipped and hit his head," the woman cries as you approach. "He's bleeding and won't wake up!"

"Kelly," you say into your portable radio as you kneel next to the teenager, "I need you to call 911 for a fall with possible head injury."

THE EMS SYSTEM

Nearly all corners of the nation are served by some form of an **emergency medical services (EMS)** system. An EMS system is a formalized system of highly trained individuals and specialized resources designed to respond to, care for, and transport victims of sudden injury and illness. EMS systems include sophisticated communications systems; ambulances (▼ Figure 1.2), helicopters, hospitals, fire and police resources; and a variety of skilled individuals who make the whole system function.

1.1 Identify the common components of an emergency medical services (EMS) system.

emergency medical services (EMS) a formalized system of highly trained individuals and specialized resources designed to respond to, care for, and transport victims of sudden injury and illness.

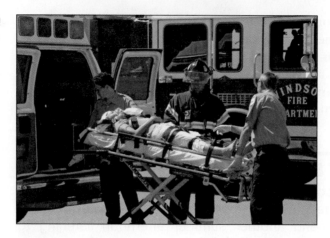

Figure 1.2 The EMS system includes a variety of resources, including ambulances and fire personnel.

Levels of Care

1.2 Differentiate among the four levels of EMS providers.

Most EMS systems include at least four levels of licensed or credentialed emergency medical providers. The most common of those are (▼ Figure 1.3) as follows:

- **Paramedic.** Generally the highest level of training in the prehospital setting, Paramedics can be found in nearly all areas of EMS, including ambulances, fire departments, law enforcement agencies, lifeguard teams, and helicopters. Paramedics receive training in advanced procedures and can give medications for a wide variety of medical conditions. Depending on the program, Paramedic training can run from approximately six months to two years.

- **Advanced Emergency Medical Technician (AEMT).** This level of training requires fewer hours than the Paramedic level. The AEMT is trained to provide a limited set of advanced skills and fewer medications than the Paramedic. Depending on the program, AEMT training can run from six months to one year.

- **Emergency Medical Technician (EMT).** The most common level of provider in the prehospital setting, EMTs can be found in nearly all areas of EMS. In most cases, EMTs are trained to provide basic life-support skills, which may include a very limited list of medications. EMT training can run from an accelerated three-week program to a year-long program.

- **Emergency Medical Responder (EMR).** The EMR requires the least amount of training in the prehospital setting and typically involves between 50 and 100 hours of training. In most systems, EMRs can provide basic life-support skills, including the use of an automated external defibrillator.

Figure 1.3 The four levels of EMS training.

Levels of EMS Training
Paramedic
Advanced EMT
Emergency Medical Technician (EMT)
Emergency Medical Responder

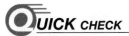

QUICK CHECK

What is the highest level of EMS training for the individual who can be found in ambulances, fire engines, and helicopters across the nation? ●

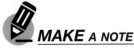

MAKE A NOTE

EMS systems can differ from state to state and region to region. The better you understand the EMS system in your area, the better you will be at using it efficiently. Take some time to discover the level of training the members of the EMS system in your area have. Is your area served by Paramedics or EMTs? Is there an EMS helicopter serving your region? Where is the nearest trauma center? ●

Pre-EMS Levels of Care

It is widely accepted that early recognition of a medical emergency combined with the prompt delivery of first-aid care can make a difference between life and death, in recovery time, and between temporary and permanent disability.[3] EMS is an intricate system of coordinated resources designed to deliver just such emergency medical care.[4] The EMS system of care begins with those who are first to recognize that an emergency exists and provide life-supporting care and appropriate first aid.[5] First aid is the emergency care provided for sudden injury or illness before care from more highly trained EMS personnel is available.

The first-aid provider in the workplace—the Emergency Responder—is someone who is trained in the delivery of initial medical emergency procedures. First-aid providers use a limited amount of equipment to perform a primary assessment and lifesaving interventions while awaiting the arrival of EMS personnel. Unlike a bystander or "passerby" who is coincidentally confronted by a fellow citizen in need and who may or may not choose to provide assistance, those with an occupational requirement to be first-aid trained may be *expected* to provide care until EMS personnel arrive.

In addition to basic first-aid training, those expected to render first aid as part of their job duties typically receive training in cardiopulmonary resuscitation (CPR), automated external defibrillation (AED), and occupational exposure to bloodborne pathogens. This initial training rarely exceeds a total of eight or nine hours. For some first-aid providers at work, this is simply not enough.

Federal officials recognized there was a gap between basic first-aid training and the training of EMS providers in the early 1970s. Their solution was *Crash Injury Management: Emergency Medical Services for Traffic Law*

---

[3]Occupational Safety and Health Administration, *Best Practices Guide: Fundamentals of a Workplace First-Aid Program.* OSHA 3317–06N 2006 (Washington, DC: U.S. Department of Labor, 2006), 5. Also available online at http://www.osha.gov/Publications/OSHA3317first-aid.pdf (accessed January 10, 2010).

[4]National Highway Traffic Safety Administration, *What Is EMS?* (Washington, DC: National Highway Traffic Safety Administration, n.d.), http://www.ems.gov/portal/site/ems/menuitem. 5149822b03938f65a8de25f076ac8789/?vgnextoid=9990f44e90578110VgnVCM1000002fd17898RCRD (accessed January 10, 2010).

[5]National Association of EMS Educators, *Pre-EMS Education and Instructor Development: Prehospital Emergency Care* 8 (2004): 319–21.

Enforcement Officers.[6] This was a standardized course designed to provide training in emergency medical care and was considered advanced first-aid training. The original intent of filling the knowledge and skill gap between basic first-aid training and EMS is the intent of the text you are reading now.

Your role as an Emergency Responder is vital to the well-being of the ill or injured person. If it were not for you, many people would have to wait far too long for help, a wait that can prove disabling or deadly.

Role of the Emergency Responder

1.3 Differentiate among the roles and responsibilities of the Emergency Responder from other EMS providers.

It is likely that your primary job is not about providing medical care to those in need (▼ Figure 1.4). If it were, you would likely be an EMS or health-care professional. As a result, it is no small task for you to step out of your normal work duties to provide emergency medical care. However, providing emergency care is only one of the many responsibilities of an Emergency Responder.

Safety Advocate

1.4 Explain the role that the Emergency Responder plays in ensuring the safety of all people at the scene of an emergency.

Emergency Responders are safety advocates in that they help ensure the safety of the public, customers, employees, visitors, and other people in the workplace. Emergency Responders are "champions" of health and safety and help to promote injury and illness prevention in the workplace. In addition to helping

Figure 1.4 For most Emergency Responders, providing medical care is not the primary duty.

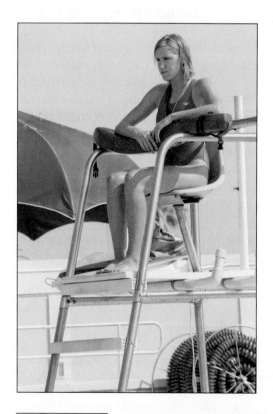

[6]National Highway Traffic Safety Administration, *Crash Injury Management: Emergency Medical Services for Traffic Law Enforcement Officers. Instructor's Lesson Plans.* DOT HS 820 283 (Washington, DC: National Highway Traffic Safety Administration, 1973). Abstract of the program plus copies of the components of the program are available at ERIC (Education Resources Information Center): http://www.eric.ed.gov/

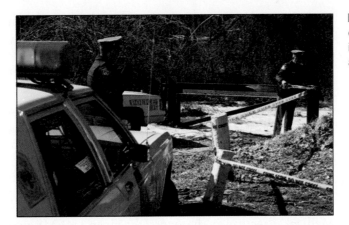

manage on-site emergencies, Emergency Responders can help to enhance relationships with public safety agencies and others within their community.

The primary responsibility of an Emergency Responder is to ensure that the scene is safe for all those who may be responding, as well as bystanders who may enter the scene unaware of any hazards (▲ Figure 1.5). Safety will be discussed in more detail throughout this book, but just know for now that you should never be expected to care for ill or injured people if it is not safe to do so. In some cases your job simply may be to keep others from entering the scene or to help make the scene safe.

Advocate for the Ill and Injured

As an Emergency Responder, it is your responsibility to be an advocate for the ill or injured person. In times of illness or injury, a person can become confused and unsure of the extent of the problem. You must remain objective and provide guidance to the ill or injured to help ensure they receive the most appropriate care.

It is not uncommon for people who have suffered an illness or injury to tell you that calling 911 is unnecessary. It may be up to you to make decisions on their behalf when they may not be fully aware of the extent of their illness or injury. Administration of first aid should not delay activation of the EMS system when required. You should activate EMS or your occupational emergency action plan immediately when any person is unresponsive, badly hurt, looks or acts very ill.

Certain minor illnesses and injuries that can be treated with first aid may not require EMS involvement or assistance by other medical professionals. However, if you are in doubt about the seriousness of the person's condition, it is usually in the best interest of all to call 911.

Lifelong Learner

Just as you must constantly be learning to stay on top of your game with your primary job, keeping up to date with your emergency care knowledge and skills is just as important. There may be long periods of time between emergency calls, when all is going well and there is no need for your emergency care knowledge or skills, but just when you least expect it, you may be called to the scene of an emergency and be expected to perform swiftly and

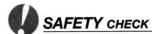

SAFETY CHECK

The most important responsibility of the Emergency Responder is to ensure the safety of all those on the scene, foremost yourself. In some cases, the ill or injured person cannot be cared for until all hazards have been appropriately addressed. Most of the common hazards, such as exposure to blood, can be easily managed without delaying care to the ill or injured person. ●

appropriately. This only can happen smoothly if you make it a practice to refresh your knowledge and practice your skills whenever possible.

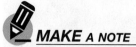

MAKE *A* **NOTE**

You might be interested to know that the services of a Medical Director were used in the development of this textbook. His familiarity with emergency medicine, EMS systems, and workplace emergency teams ensures that only current and accurate practice is presented in this textbook. ●

Medical Direction

1.6 Explain the concept of medical direction and how it relates to the Emergency Responder.

medical direction the oversight given to EMS providers by a physician.

Medical Director the physician in charge of an EMS system.

protocols emergency care guidelines developed in cooperation with the Medical Director; they provide EMS personnel and some Emergency Responders with recommended procedures for emergency care.

Medical direction is the oversight given to EMS providers by a physician. The physician in charge of an EMS system is called the **Medical Director**. Physician medical direction is a requirement of all EMS systems. Even though you may not be working within a formal EMS system, your organization or agency may have a Medical Director. As an Emergency Responder, you may never have a reason to interact directly with your Medical Director, but you may interact indirectly by way of predefined emergency action plans, organizational policies, or emergency response guidelines.

Guidelines for providing emergency medical care are sometimes referred to as **protocols** and are developed in cooperation with a Medical Director. In the absence of formal emergency medical care protocols in your workplace, you should provide emergency care based on the training you receive in this program. All workplaces should have an emergency action plan (EAP) that describes how to notify designated first-aid providers in an emergency and clarifies what is expected of them when they respond. The plan should include the preferred means for alerting EMS from the worksite and for helping EMS get to the ill or injured person. Putting together a comprehensive EAP involves evaluating the specific worksite layout, structural features, and emergency systems.

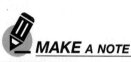

MAKE *A* **NOTE**

The U.S. Department of Labor's Occupational Safety and Health Administration (OSHA) has a helpful EAP Web site available at http://www.osha.gov/SLTC/etools/evacuation/eap.html. ●

ACCESSING EMS

1.5 Explain the various methods used to access the EMS system.

At the core of all EMS systems is the 911 access number. In North America, 911 is the universal access number for all fire, police, and EMS resources. Emergency services can be accessed by dialing 911 from a landline such as a house phone, work phone, or pay phone. A cell phone also can be used to access 911. Individuals working in public safety, emergency management, public health, and public works, typically use radio systems to activate EMS. However, when you have a choice between a cell phone and a landline, it is preferred that you use a landline to access 911, because it is more likely to be directed to a local dispatch center (▶ Figure 1.6). Also, in many 911 systems,

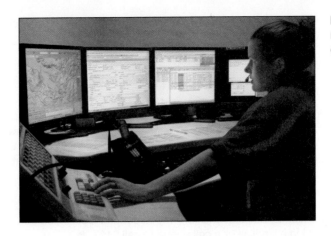

Figure 1.6 A 911 dispatcher receives calls from many different sources.

the dispatcher will be able to identify the location of the caller and the number he is calling from.

Another common method for accessing the 911 system is through the use of a highway call box. Call boxes typically have cellular-style phones that provide a direct connection to the appropriate dispatch center. Call boxes are located at fixed positions along a highway, so the dispatcher always knows where the caller is located.

In some workplaces or industrial settings, dialing 911 from your work phone may not be so easy. Many of the phone systems in workplace settings require that you dial a specific number, such as 9, to obtain an outside line before you can successfully make a 911 call (▼ Figure 1.7). It is important to

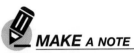

MAKE _A NOTE_

Most standard phone lines are answered by a local EMS dispatcher. However, a 911 call made from a cell phone may be answered by a dispatcher miles away in a different town or county. You must always be prepared to state your exact location when making a 911 call from a cell phone. ●

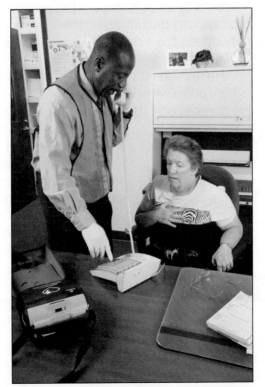

Figure 1.7 You must be familiar with the most efficient means of activating your emergency action plan and 911.

thoroughly understand your occupational emergency plan, including the requirements to activate EMS in your environment, so that you do not inadvertently cause a delay.

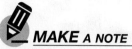

MAKE A NOTE

At many large work and industrial sites, the first responders are security officers and/or emergency response teams trained in emergency care. In these environments, there often is a dedicated internal number or announcement code that is used to activate them. ●

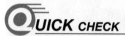

QUICK CHECK

Which is the most efficient way to contact local resources in the event of an emergency—using a landline or a cell phone to call 911? ●

THE HANDOFF

"I need you to put your hands here and here," you say as you instruct the bystander to hold the patient's head in a neutral, in-line position. "Hold his head firmly and keep it straight, just like that, okay?"

"Um, okay." The man looks nervous but continues stabilizing the patient's head and spine properly.

You place your ear close to the patient's mouth and listen carefully, relieved to hear slow, steady breathing. You reassure the panicked woman and further encourage the man holding the patient's head as you put on gloves and pull a thick gauze pad from the response bag, placing it onto the steadily bleeding wound toward the back of the injured boy's head.

You are just reaching for the portable radio again when you hear sirens approaching quickly from the direction of the highway. Within minutes, Kelly opens the side gate and leads an ambulance crew through into the pool area.

"He fell and hit the back of his head on the concrete," you say to EMTs as they pull a wheeled stretcher to you. "He's been unresponsive for about five minutes now, but he's been breathing steadily. I've also got the bleeding controlled."

With a rush of communication and activity, the boy is strapped to a backboard and placed onto the stretcher. After thanking you for your quick actions, the EMTs disappear through the open gate, leaving you standing in the murmuring crowd, hoping the outcome will be good for the boy and grateful that your emergency care knowledge and skills helped you play a positive role in this tragic event.

CHAPTER REVIEW

Chapter Summary

- EMS systems are made up of many components, such as hospitals, ambulances, dispatch centers, fire departments, and specially trained personnel who work together to respond to, care for, and transport victims of sudden illness and injury.

- Commonly, there is a minimum of four levels of field provider training in an EMS system: Paramedic, Advanced Emergency Medical Technician (AEMT), Emergency Medical Technician (EMT), and Emergency Medical Responder (EMR).

- The EMS system of care begins with those who are first to recognize that an emergency exists and to apply accepted principles of life-supporting care until EMS personnel arrive. This is the role of the Emergency Responder.

- One of the primary responsibilities of emergency responders is to ensure safety for themselves as well as others at the scene.

- In the United States, the EMS system is activated by calling 911 from a landline telephone, such as a house phone, work phone, or pay phone. A cell phone or highway call box can also be used to access 911.

- All EMS systems must have a physician who serves as a Medical Director. It is his or her responsibility to oversee the training and care delivered by field personnel. As an Emergency Responder, you do not fall under the jurisdiction of the EMS medical director, but the business, agency, or institution for which you work may have a physician serving as Medical Director.

Quick Quiz

1. Which one of the following is *not* a component of a typical EMS system?

   a. Ambulance service

   b. Rehabilitation center

   c. Hospital

   d. Communication center

2. Which level of EMS provider is the most common and is trained to provide basic life-support care as well as transport people to a hospital?

   a. Paramedic

   b. Advanced EMT

   c. EMT

   d. EMR

3. As an Emergency Responder, your primary responsibility at the scene of an emergency is to:

   a. activate 911.

   b. quickly assess the ill or injured person.

   c. ensure that the scene is safe.

   d. move the ill or injured person to safety.

4. In the EMS system, the _____ is the person responsible for developing emergency care protocols.

   a. EMS provider

   b. Paramedic

   c. chief officer

   d. Medical Director

5. In the workplace, it is usually better to access 911 using a:

   a. cell phone.

   b. land line.

   c. pager.

   d. highway call box.

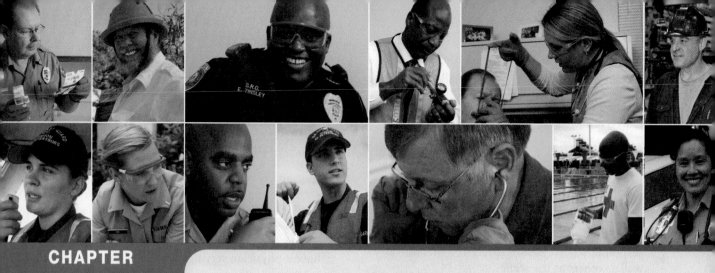

Legal and Ethical Principles of Emergency Care

KEY TERMS

The following terms are introduced in this chapter:

- abandonment *(p. 16)*
- advance directive *(p. 19)*
- battery *(p. 18)*
- breach of duty *(p. 16)*
- confidentiality *(p. 14)*
- consent *(p. 16)*
- duty of care *(p. 16)*
- ethics *(p. 13)*
- expressed consent *(p. 16)*
- Good Samaritan laws *(p. 15)*
- implied consent *(p. 17)*
- mandated reporter *(p. 19)*
- mentally competent *(p. 17)*
- negligence *(p. 17)*

LEARNING OBJECTIVES

At the conclusion of this chapter and the associated instructor-guided lesson, the student will be able to:

Cognitive

2.1 Define the term *ethics* and how it relates to the Emergency Responder. *(p. 13)*

2.2 Explain the role of the Emergency Responder with regards to confidentiality. *(p. 14)*

2.3 Explain the term *Good Samaritan laws* and how these laws relate to the Emergency Responder. *(p. 15)*

2.4 Explain the concepts of *duty of care* and *breach of duty* as they relate to the Emergency Responder. *(p. 16)*

2.5 Define the term *consent* and the various types of consent utilized by the Emergency Responder. *(p. 16)*

2.6 Explain the role of the Emergency Responder for ill or injured people who refuse care. *(p. 18)*

2.7 Define the following terms and the role of the Emergency Responder with each: *abandonment, negligence,* and *battery*. *(p. 17)*

2.8 Define the term *mandated reporter* and how it relates to the Emergency Responder. *(p. 19)*

2.9 Explain the common elements of an advance directive. *(p. 19)*

2.10 Explain the role of the Emergency Responder when confronted with an advance directive. *(p. 19)*

Introduction

*I*T is truly commendable that you have chosen to be a part of a unique set of individuals who willingly respond when others are in need. This is no easy task. You may be a law enforcement officer, firefighter, lifeguard, security officer, or part of a corporate or industrial emergency response team, which means you have a primary job that you must do each and every day. If this last scenario is the case, the part of your job that now requires you to respond to and assist at the scene of a medical emergency is only a small part of your overall responsibilities. Be assured that this text takes that into consideration and aims to do everything possible to prepare you for this role.

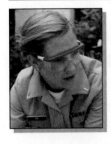

THE EMERGENCY

You are on a routine vehicle patrol in the city's north side, a vast maze of winding residential neighborhoods and boxlike strip malls, when you see an older man suddenly lurch forward off a bus stop bench and fall to the sidewalk. You contact dispatch on your squad car's radio and request a medical response to the location as you pull across both lanes, parking near the curb with your light bar pulsing.

You grab the response bag from your trunk, pull on a pair of purple exam gloves, and kneel next to the man, who is blinking rapidly and trying to sit up. "Just relax, sir," you say. "I'm trained in emergency medical care. Is it okay if I help you?"

"No," the man pushes your hand away. "I'm fine. I was feeling a little woozy and I think I blacked out for a minute, but I'm okay now."

"Sir, I really think it would be better if you at least stay where you are until the ambulance gets here." You can hear the sirens several blocks away.

"I don't need an ambulance." He pulls himself back up onto the bench and sits, breathing rapidly. "And I told you that I don't want any help!"

"I get it," you say, sitting next to the man and setting the nylon bag between your feet. "I probably wouldn't want help if I were you."

"Really?" He looks at you, eyebrows raised.

THE ETHICS OF BEING AN EMERGENCY RESPONDER

Ethics is the study of the principles (rules) that define behavior as right, good, and proper. As an Emergency Responder, you will be making a commitment to assist an injured or ill person who is in need. This is no small task. Accepting the roles and responsibilities of an Emergency Responder means that you must apply your emergency care knowledge and skills to the best of your ability. You also must remain committed to continual training in order to keep your knowledge and skills fresh and ready when you need them. The people you will be caring for expect it and depend on it.

2.1 Define the term *ethics* and how it relates to the Emergency Responder.

ethics the study of the principles (rules) that define behavior as right, good, and proper.

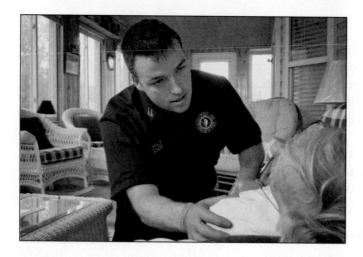

Figure 2.1 One of the most important skills an Emergency Responder can possess is compassion.

ADVOCACY FOR THE ILL AND INJURED

A very important ethical aspect related to caring for ill and injured people is the concept of advocacy. As an Emergency Responder, you must be an advocate for them. In short, this means putting their needs before your own (as long as it is safe to do so).

The word *advocate* literally means to "speak in favor of" or "plead in another's behalf" (▲ Figure 2.1). Ill or injured people are often distracted by and may even be confused by what is happening to them. They depend on you to consider what is best given their circumstances. They must rely on you to assist them in making the most appropriate decisions regarding the care that they need. Don't worry. In most cases it will be relatively obvious what the person needs, and in many situations you will have other Emergency Responders to help in the decision-making process. When in doubt, call 911.

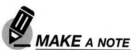

MAKE *A NOTE*

As an Emergency Responder, it is sometimes challenging to do what is right for ill or injured people because they may not be willing to accept the care that you are offering. Their refusal may be influenced by their illness or injury or other concerns. However, just because they refuse care initially does not mean you can stop being their advocate. When in doubt, consult with others on your team or consider calling 911 and allowing the EMS providers to evaluate the person. ●

CONFIDENTIALITY

2.2 Explain the role of the Emergency Responder with regards to confidentiality.

confidentiality the obligation not to share information about an event or a person's condition with anyone except those who are directly involved in the incident or the person's care.

Being injured or experiencing a sudden illness is a very personal matter. To an Emergency Responder, it often means seeing people when they are at their worst and in a very vulnerable state, both physically and emotionally. As a result, you have an ethical obligation to respect their privacy and maintain a high degree of **confidentiality** (▶ Figure 2.2).

Maintaining confidentiality means that you will share information about the event or the person's condition only with those directly involved in his

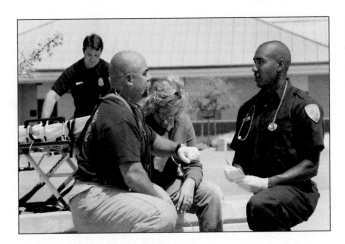

Figure 2.2 Sharing of information with those who take over emergency care of the patient is a necessary and important part of good patient care.

care. It is legal and appropriate to share information with other care providers, such as EMS personnel, hospital personnel, or others who are directly involved in the care of the ill or injured person.

LEGAL ASPECTS OF PROVIDING CARE

There are legal aspects of emergency care that you must be aware of as an Emergency Responder. Among others, they include issues of liability, duty, consent, and advance directives.

2.3 Explain the term *Good Samaritan law* and how these laws relate to the Emergency Responder.

Good Samaritan Laws

Good Samaritan laws exist in all 50 states. They are designed to encourage passersby to stop and render care to an ill or injured person by limiting the exposure to civil liability. In most cases, Good Samaritan laws only protect people who are rendering care without an expectation of payment for services rendered. That includes physicians, nurses, firefighters, and any other Emergency Responder, unless they act in a reckless or grossly negligent manner. The Good Samaritan laws do not apply to health-care providers who are providing emergency medical care as part of their normal job, such as an EMT or Paramedic responding in an ambulance.

Good Samaritan laws laws existing in all 50 states designed to encourage "passersby" to stop and render care to an ill or injured person by limiting the exposure to civil liability.

Providing that the Emergency Responder acts in good faith and within the limits of his training, and not recklessly or in a grossly negligent manner, it is very unlikely that legal action would be taken against an Emergency Responder who is designated or expected by his employer to provide first aid in an emergency. However, if you are concerned about liability as a designated first-aid provider at work, you should speak with your employer. It is very possible that you would be covered by your employer's insurance in your capacity as an Emergency Responder.

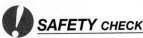 **SAFETY** *CHECK*

Even though Good Samaritan laws are designed to encourage Emergency Responders to stop to assist those in need, you are not expected to do so if the scene is unsafe. Your highest priority is always your own safety as well as the safety of others at the scene. ●

duty of care the responsibility to others to act according to the law.

Duty of Care

Duty of care is the requirement that a person act toward others and the public with the watchfulness, attention, caution, and prudence that a reasonable person in similar circumstances would use. If a person's actions do not meet this standard, then the acts may be considered negligent, and any damages resulting may be claimed in a lawsuit for negligence.

Usually, public safety professionals, such as law enforcement or EMS personnel, responding to an emergency call have a legal duty to render care to an ill or injured person. However, state occupational licensing regulations vary widely and may impose a duty of care on first-aid providers as well. If you are required to meet state licensing regulations in your occupation, it is imperative that you be completely familiar with those regulations. If you are an Emergency Responder who is designated or expected by your employer to provide first aid in an emergency (for example, as part of an occupational emergency medical response team), it is best to assume that you have a legal duty to act.

breach of duty a legal term referring to the occasion when someone who has a duty to provide care fails to do so.

abandonment a legal term for leaving an ill or injured person before an equal or more highly trained person can assume responsibility for care.

If you have a legal duty to render care and fail to do so, or do so in a reckless or grossly negligent manner, you could be considered in **breach of duty** and found legally liable. Ways in which you can breach a duty to act is simply to fail to provide appropriate care. Another possible breach of duty could occur if you were to leave an ill or injured person before someone with equal or higher training took over care. This is commonly referred to as **abandonment**.

Now, do not let this discussion about the legal aspects of providing emergency care discourage you. As long as you act in good faith and within the limits of your training, it is very unlikely that your care will ever come into question. Always using good common sense and at all times keeping the best interest of the ill or injured person in mind make up the foundation of good care.

Obtaining Consent

consent permission to provide care.

expressed consent a type of consent that occurs when a conscious person gives permission for care.

It is important for an Emergency Responder to obtain permission from the ill or injured person before beginning care. This permission is called **consent**, and it can take several forms. The most common type of consent is called **expressed consent**. This occurs when you ask a conscious person for permission to care for him and he agrees to that care. Expressed consent is sometimes called "informed consent."

Obtaining consent is one of the very first things you will want to do before you begin caring for an ill or injured person and can be a part of your introduction. For instance, as you come up to the person, you might say something like, "Hello, my name is Chris. I am a member of the company emergency response team. May I help you?" In most instances the person will respond with a yes. You now have gained consent and may begin providing emergency care.

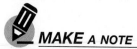

MAKE A NOTE

Expressed consent can be verbal, nonverbal, or written. A conscious person may not be able to speak, but his actions can indicate that he wants you to help him. As long as it is reasonable to think that he understands that you are there to assist and he does not resist your efforts to help, an action such as a nod can be viewed as informed consent. ●

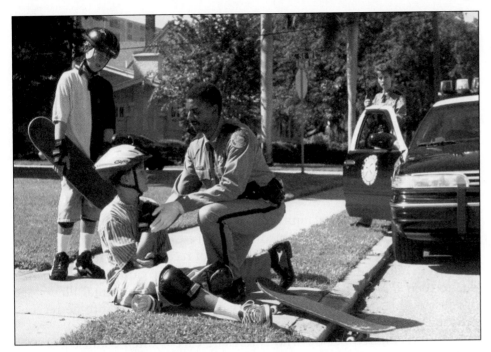

PEDIATRIC CARE

In most circumstances, a minor cannot legally consent to or refuse care. A parent or legal guardian must do so. When a parent or guardian is not available, you may provide care based on a legal concept referred to as "implied consent." It is implied that if the parent or guardian had knowledge of the situation, he or she would consent to care for the child. ●

Implied Consent

Keep in mind that the ability to grant legal consent only applies to people of legal age. For instance, a 10-year-old child does not have the legal right either to grant consent for care or to refuse care. As an Emergency Responder, you can legally begin care for minors based on the concept of **implied consent**. It is implied that if the parents or guardians knew of their child's condition, they would grant consent for care (▲ Figure 2.3).

    Perhaps you are wondering what to do if an ill or injured person is unconscious. The concept of consent still applies. You may be able to begin care on the basis of "implied consent." Implied consent allows you to care for someone who is not conscious because it is assumed that if the unconscious person were conscious and alert, he would give you consent to care for him.

implied consent a form of consent used for unconscious people or people under the legal age of consent.

Mental Competency

In addition to being over the age of 18, a person also must be **mentally competent** to legally grant consent. This can get a little tricky, but just understand that people who are under the influence of drugs or alcohol, or who are so badly injured that they do not fully understand their condition, may not be competent to refuse care. When in doubt about a person's ability to make good decisions in this regard, provide emergency care as the circumstances reasonably allow. Activate your emergency action plan or call 911. Let the EMS professionals take over when they arrive.

mentally competent refers to people who are of sound mind and judgment and are able to make appropriate decisions about their own medical care.

2.7 Define the following terms and the role of the Emergency Responder with each: *abandonment, negligence,* and *battery.*

Negligence

Negligence is defined as failure to exercise care toward others that a reasonable or prudent person would in the same circumstances or failure to take

negligence failure to exercise the care toward others that a reasonable or prudent person would in the same circumstance.

action that a reasonable person would take. As an Emergency Responder, you are expected to provide prudent and reasonable care at all times, provide care that is within the limits of your training, and do nothing that would further harm the ill or injured person.

Many of the concepts mentioned next—such as abandonment, battery, and providing care outside of the limits of your training—could all be considered grounds for negligence. Using good common sense and keeping the best interest of the ill or injured person in mind at all times will go a long way in preventing claims of negligence.

Refusal of Care

2.6 Explain the role of the Emergency Responder for ill or injured people who refuse care.

Surprisingly, not all ill or injured people want someone to care for them. There are many reasons why someone may refuse care including but not limited to religious beliefs, terminal illness, fear of receiving a large bill, and fear of pain. In addition, ill or injured people who refuse care may be impaired due to their injury or illness, or from drugs, alcohol, or mental illness. Do not just dismiss them. Leaving an ill or injured person before he receives proper care could be considered abandonment.

An ill or injured person who is refusing care is often confused, scared, and embarrassed all at once. This is a time to be as calm and reassuring as you can and do your best to listen to his or her concerns. Encourage the person to seek more advanced medical care.

There is no legal duty to provide unwanted treatment. You are not legally permitted to force care on anyone. Attempting to restrain or force care onto someone could be considered **battery**.

battery a legal term for forcing care on someone who does not want it.

In many cases, when you arrive on scene, someone has already activated the emergency action plan or called 911. In this situation, your job will be to listen calmly to the person and try to persuade him or her to be evaluated by EMS. Many ill or injured people are more willing to listen to someone in a uniform, and EMS providers are usually quite skilled at convincing people that it is "better to be safe than sorry" and at least be evaluated by a physician.

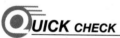 **UICK** *CHECK*

When is it necessary for you to remain at the emergency scene or with the injured or ill person? ●

It is especially important to carefully document situations in which an ill or injured person refuses care. Your documentation should include what happened to the person, all of his or her complaints, signs and symptoms, and your attempts to encourage the person to seek more advanced care.

 PEDIATRIC *CARE*

Remember that a minor cannot legally refuse care. Therefore, if the minor is refusing to allow you to provide care, you must call 911 for assistance. ●

It is possible that a person you are caring for does not need more advanced care or simply insists on refusing care as any competent adult may choose to do. In these cases, if you are able, take the time to check in on the person. For example, if he is a guest or coworker, call or stop to see how he is doing.

Just remember, when things get difficult the best thing to do is call 911. EMS professionals are well versed in dealing with people who refuse care, including making sure that they understand the risks and consequences of their decision and that the refusal is properly documented.

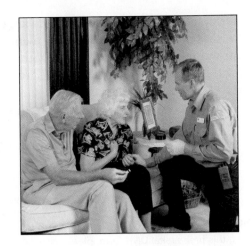

Figure 2.4 Abuse and neglect are unfortunately a common problem among the elderly.

Mandated Reporter

Another important concept that you must understand as someone who is receiving training in the care of ill and injured people is that of the **mandated reporter**. A mandated reporter is someone who is legally obligated to report any suspicion of abuse or neglect. While most often thought of as being related to children, abuse and neglect are unfortunately a common problem among the elderly as well (▲ Figure 2.4). Each state defines a mandated reporter differently, so you and your instructor will need to do a little research to discover who your state defines as mandated reporters. This is not difficult. Typing your state and "mandated reporter" into an Internet search engine should provide you the necessary links to your state requirements.

Typical roles that are frequently defined as mandated reporters are teachers, clergy, medical staff, counselors, and day care providers. While the definition of a mandated reporter may differ from state to state, the responsibilities are usually the same and very clear. A mandated reporter must immediately report any case of suspected abuse or neglect to either a law enforcement officer or child protective services. Your instructor will discuss the specifics regarding mandated reporter laws in your state.

2.8 Define the term *mandated reporter* and how it relates to the Emergency Responder.

mandated reporter a person who is legally obligated to report any suspicion of abuse or neglect.

👤 *PEDIATRIC* CARE

Know the laws in your state regarding mandated reporters. With your level of training, you may be legally required to report any suspected case of abuse or neglect. ●

Advance Directives

An **advance directive** is a legal document that outlines a person's wishes regarding his own health care. Advance directives are becoming more common as people are becoming more informed about end-of-life issues. It is quite possible that you could be called to the aid of someone who is ill or dying and you are told by caregivers or family members that the person has an advance directive. You must be informed as to what your obligations are for these situations.

One of the most common forms of an advance directive is called a "do not resuscitate" (DNR) order. A DNR is typically initiated when a person is

2.9 Explain the common elements of an advance directive.

2.10 Explain the role of the Emergency Responder when confronted with an advance directive.

advance directive a legal document that outlines a person's wishes regarding his or her own health care.

terminally ill. Not all DNR orders are the same. The orders reflect the specific wishes of the person and family members. To be valid, a DNR order must be in written form and presented with the person (▼ Figure 2.5). You may not withhold care simply because a family member tells you a loved one has a DNR. You must physically see the written order and understand what the order directs you to do or not do. In some cases it may state that there are to be no resuscitative efforts of any kind. In other cases it may state that the person wants you to provide rescue breaths and oxygen but does not want you

PREHOSPITAL DO NOT RESUSCITATE ORDERS

ATTENDING PHYSICIAN

In completing this prehospital DNR form, please check part A if no intervention by prehospital personnel is indicated. Please check Part A and options from Part B if specific interventions by prehospital personnel are indicated. To give a valid prehospital DNR order, this form must be completed by the patient's attending physician and must be provided to prehospital personnel.

A) _____ **Do Not Resuscitate (DNR):**
No Cardiopulmonary Resuscitation or Advanced Cardiac Life Support be performed by prehospital personnel

B) _____ **Modified Support:**
Prehospital personnel administer the following checked options:
_____ Oxygen administration
_____ Full airway support: intubation, airways, bag/valve/mask
_____ Venipuncture: IV crystalloids and/or blood draw
_____ External cardiac pacing
_____ Cardiopulmonary resuscitation
_____ Cardiac defibrillator
_____ Pneumatic anti-shock garment
_____ Ventilator
_____ ACLS meds
_____ Other interventions/medications (physician specify)
_____

Prehospital personnel are informed that (print patient name)_____
should receive no resuscitation (DNR) or should receive Modified Support as indicated. This directive is medically appropriate and is further documented by a physician's order and a progress note on the patient's permanent medical record. Informed consent from the capacitated patient or the incapacitated patient's legitimate surrogate is documented on the patient's permanent medical record. The DNR order is in full force and effect as of the date indicated below.

_____   _____
Attending Physician's Signature

_____   _____
Print Attending Physician's Name   Print Patient's Name and Location
                                            (Home Address or Health Care Facility)

_____
Attending Physician's Telephone

_____   _____
Date   Expiration Date (6 Mos from Signature)

Figure 2.5 A common example of a DNR order.

to begin chest compressions. Again, each DNR order is different, so you must clearly understand the directive as it pertains to the specific person.

In instances when it is unclear or uncertain if the person has a valid advance directive, it is always best to activate your emergency action plan and call 911. If it is safe to do so, initiate the appropriate care while waiting for EMS.

THE HANDOFF

"So what's going on today?" the EMT asks you, as she pulls a large red bag from the back of the ambulance.

"I was driving past and saw Mr. Murdoch here fall to the ground," you say. "He apparently wasn't feeling well and thinks he may have lost consciousness. I was able to check his vitals and get a good history while waiting for you."

She looks past you at the man and says, "Mr. Murdoch? You were able to get vitals and a history on Mr. Murdoch? How did you do that?" she asks you quietly as her partner pulls the gurney out of the ambulance with a clatter. "He normally won't even talk to us."

"I've found that a lot of times people are just scared," you say, helping to position the gurney next to Mr. Murdoch, who quickly moves himself onto it from the bench. "Acknowledging fears, building some rapport, and explaining what you are going to do and why goes a long way toward breaking down those barriers."

"You know, I'm going to try that from now on." The EMT smiles at you and then turns to the patient. "Mr. Murdoch, is it okay if we get you over to see the doctor and make sure that you're okay?"

As you watch the ambulance navigate back into traffic you smile, knowing that you may have just made a real difference for the patient and the EMT.

CHAPTER REVIEW

Chapter Summary

- Ethics is the study of the rules that define behavior as right, good, and proper. As an Emergency Responder, you have an ethical obligation to do what is right for each ill or injured person you may encounter.

- Confidentiality is a part of that ethical behavior. You must keep confidential the information that you gather when caring for ill or injured people. It is ethical and legal to share information with others who will be caring for those people.

- Good Samaritan laws exist in every state and are designed to encourage bystanders, passersby, and laypeople to stop and render care to ill or injured people by limiting their exposure to liability.

- As an Emergency Responder, you may have a legal duty to provide care when called upon to do so. Failing to respond when you have a legal duty to do so could be considered a breach of duty.

- You must obtain consent prior to beginning care. This consent can be expressed or implied, depending on the situation.

- It is not unusual for an ill or injured person to refuse care. Be extra careful in these situations and consider calling 911. Let the EMS team assist the person in making the right decision for the person's condition.

- Once you begin care for someone, you have a legal duty to remain and continue care until someone of equal or higher training takes over. Leaving the person before you are legally allowed to do so may be considered abandonment.

- Breach of duty and abandonment are just two examples of what could be considered negligence.

- You may not force care on someone who does want your help. Doing so could result in an accusation of battery.

- As an Emergency Responder trained in emergency care, you may have a legal duty to report any suspicion of abuse and neglect. This applies to both children and the elderly. Research your state laws and requirements for mandatory reporters on the Internet or with your instructor to see if your role as an Emergency Responder identifies you as a mandated reporter in your state.

- An advance directive is a legal document that outlines the medical care wishes of the ill or injured person. You are required to follow the directions specified in the person's advance directive.

Quick Quiz

1. The term that refers to your legal obligation to assist an ill or injured person is:
   a. obligatory.
   b. duty.
   c. necessity.
   d. advocacy.

2. As an Emergency Responder, you are not to discuss information about the ill or injured person with others unless they are directly involved with the person's care. This is known as:
   a. duty.
   b. breach of duty.
   c. confidentiality.
   d. ethics.

3. You are allowed to care for an unconscious person who is injured based on _____ consent.
   a. expressed
   b. informed
   c. applied
   d. implied

4. You are caring for an ill person who becomes unconscious. You get overwhelmed and decide to leave the scene. You may be accused of a negligent act called:
   a. abandonment.
   b. battery.
   c. duty.
   d. advocacy.

5. Which one of the following is the most appropriate way to manage an ill or injured person who you feel is in need of care but is refusing it?
   a. Leave your number and direct him to call if things get worse.
   b. Call 911.
   c. Report him to his supervisor.
   d. Have him sign a release of liability form.

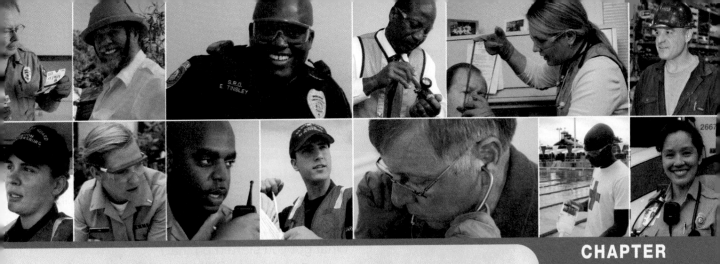

The Wellness and Safety of the Emergency Responder

LEARNING OBJECTIVES

At the conclusion of this chapter and the associated instructor-guided lesson, the student will be able to:

Cognitive

3.1 Describe common hazards at the scene of an emergency. *(p. 24)*

3.2 Describe steps the Emergency Responder should take to mitigate common scene hazards. *(p. 25)*

3.3 Identify the four routes that pathogens use to enter the body. *(p. 26)*

3.4 Define the term *standard precautions* and how it relates to the Emergency Responder. *(p. 27)*

3.5 Define body substance isolation (BSI) precautions and when they should be used. *(p. 27)*

3.6 List examples of personal protective equipment and the purpose of each. *(p. 27)*

3.7 Explain the procedure the Emergency Responder should follow after a possible exposure. *(p. 29)*

3.8 Differentiate between cleaning and disinfection, and state when each should be performed. *(p. 29)*

3.9 Define the terms *stress* and *stressor* as they relate to the Emergency Responder. *(p. 29)*

3.10 Describe several sources of stressors commonly encountered by the Emergency Responder. *(p. 30)*

3.11 Describe common physical, emotional, and behavioral responses to stress. *(p. 30)*

3.12 Describe strategies for minimizing the affects of stress on the Emergency Responder. *(p. 31)*

Psychomotor

3.13 Demonstrate proper hand-washing techniques, including use of soap and water and alcohol-based hand rubs.

3.14 Demonstrate the proper application and removal of personal protective equipment.

KEY TERMS

The following terms are introduced in this chapter:

- body substance isolation (BSI) precautions *(p. 27)*
- critical incident stress *(p. 30)*
- exposure *(p. 26)*
- pathogen *(p. 26)*
- personal protective equipment *(p. 27)*
- standard precautions *(p. 27)*
- stress *(p. 30)*
- stressor *(p. 30)*

Introduction

RESPONDING to the needs of an ill or injured person can be very stressful, especially when it is not your primary job function. This chapter addresses some of the more common sources of stress you are likely to encounter, such as personal safety and emotional and physical well-being.

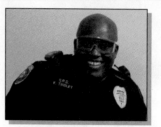

THE EMERGENCY

"I hear you took up jogging," Roger says, leaning against the counter in the spacious Fire Station 6 kitchen, where you are busily preparing a salad. "What got you started on that?"

"I was talking to Beth over at Station 3 a few weeks ago," you say. "And she was telling me how exercising and eating healthy are two great ways to prepare for the stress of this job."

"And we all know how much you like to be prepared." Roger smiles and playfully takes one of the small, red tomatoes from the salad bowl before walking out of the kitchen.

Just then, the station house fills with the electronic blare of dispatch tones, followed by an amplified voice summoning your team to a vehicle collision on Burke Avenue, one block south of the elementary school. You slide the salad into the refrigerator, hurry to the truck bay, and feel your heart beginning to beat faster as you pull on your turnouts.

"Control says a kid got hit by one of the cars." Roger climbs up into the truck and drops heavily into the seat next to you. "I hate responding to calls with kids, you know?"

You nod, your stomach tightening as you anticipate what you might encounter as the fire engine pulls from the station and rolls off toward Burke Avenue.

SAFETY FIRST

3.1 Describe common hazards at the scene of an emergency.

Emergency scenes can present a wide variety of hazards for Emergency Responders and bystanders alike. Emergency scenes that involve motor vehicles can present a laundry list of hazards, both immediate and potential, for anyone who enters the scene in an attempt to help those in need. Sharp metal, broken glass, spilled fuel, and unstable vehicles are just a few of the factors that can cause serious injury to anyone working in or around the vehicles (▶ Figure 3.1). And if that list is not enough to think about, there is the vehicle traffic that may be trying to navigate around the collision scene while you are struggling to help those who are injured.

Emergency scenes that involve explosions, fire, or hazardous chemicals can pose a risk for those located near and far from the scene. Confined spaces such as enclosed rooms, underground vaults, and large storage containers all pose a risk that is likely to be invisible (a low-oxygen environment). Catastrophic natural disasters such as hurricanes and man-made disasters such as mass shootings can put you and others at significant risk.

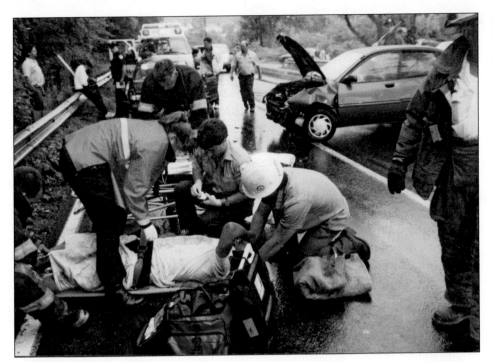

 SAFETY CHECK

Safety must always be your top priority. Resist the urge to rush into any emergency scene. You must first stop and observe the entire scene to identify any immediate or potential hazards. Only after you have determined it is safe to do so, enter the scene and begin caring for the ill or injured. ●

Minimizing Risk

Your personal safety is your top priority at every emergency scene, period! This cannot be said enough, and in fact you will see this message many times throughout this book. Trained EMS personnel get this drilled into their heads at all levels of training because it is the key to a successful career as an EMS professional. On the other hand, you may not have the benefit of continuous training, so make sure you understand that your safety is *the* top priority.

3.2 Describe steps the Emergency Responder should take to mitigate common scene hazards.

To put it another way, no matter what your level of training or experience, you have no obligation to help an ill or injured person if it puts you at significant risk of harm. You have an obligation to do your best to mitigate obvious hazards before entering the scene, as long as you can do so safely. Making the scene safe before you enter not only makes it less likely that you will be harmed, it also makes it less likely that those arriving after you will be harmed.

 MAKE A NOTE

You will never be expected to help another person if it puts you at an unreasonable risk. Your primary responsibility is to ensure your own safety, the safety of others at the scene, and the safety of the ill or injured person. Responding without concern for safety is reckless and unacceptable. ●

To understand how you might be able to mitigate a hazard, you must first learn the types of hazards that could exist at various scenes, such as the ones mentioned above. Next, you must understand your limitations with what you can and cannot do about mitigating hazards. Take a traffic collision scene as an example, assuming that the collision occurred on a somewhat busy stretch of road. You could pull to the side of the road and when there is a break in traffic, dart out to one of the damaged vehicles. This would be very dangerous and the result could be life threatening. If you were thinking about safety, your first step in making the scene safe would be to alert oncoming traffic and attempt to get the drivers to slow down. Turning on your vehicle flashers, placing flares a distance from the scene, and even alerting oncoming traffic by waving your arms are all ways to alert unsuspecting drivers that a hazard exists. Public and private safety, security, and service personnel, as well as members of business emergency response teams, all must be familiar with and follow safety and emergency procedures outlined in their emergency action plans. Bottom line: Your safety is your first priority.

It is important to resist rushing into any emergency scene, because it is much more likely to result in injury to you or others. A helpful tool for remembering what to do before entering the scene of an emergency is the acronym SETUP:

QUICK CHECK

Is it ever appropriate to help another person if it puts you at an unreasonable risk? ●

S – *Stop*. Stand still and observe the scene for all hazards.

E – *Environment*. Observe the surroundings and look for any environmental hazards.

T – *Traffic*. Look for any oncoming traffic and take steps to alert drivers that a hazard exists.

U – *Unknown hazard*. Keep an eye out for potential hazards or ones that are not immediately obvious.

P – *Protect yourself and the ill or injured person*. Use appropriate barriers to protect yourself from exposure to blood or possible diseases. These barriers also help to protect the person in your care as well.

Beware of Pathogens

3.3 Identify the four routes that pathogens use to enter the body.

pathogens germs that can cause disease.

exposure the condition of being subjected to a fluid or substance capable of transmitting an infectious agent in a manner that may have a harmful effect.

One of most common hazards when caring for any ill or injured person is the possibility of exposure to a disease-causing germ. Germs that can cause disease are referred to as **pathogens**, and everyone has the potential to carry and spread pathogens. Pathogens can be spread from person to person, and some of the most dangerous pathogens are carried in the blood. For this reason, you must minimize your risk of exposure when caring for ill or injured people. An **exposure** is the condition of being subjected to a fluid or substance capable of transmitting an infectious agent in a manner that may have a harmful effect.

Pathogens can enter the body in one or more of the following ways:

- **Ingestion.** This occurs when we eat or swallow something that is contaminated with pathogens or otherwise harmful to our health.

- **Inhalation.** This occurs when we breathe in fumes, vapors, or airborne particles that contain disease-causing pathogens.

- **Absorption.** This occurs when pathogens are allowed to be absorbed through contact with the skin.
- **Injection.** This can occur when someone is poked or stuck with a contaminated needle or sharp object.

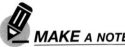

MAKE A NOTE

Being exposed to a person's blood or body fluids is a risk, but that risk is easily mitigated by taking proper precautions, such as wearing gloves, a facemask, and eye protection. In most situations you can easily and safely care for an ill or injured person when proper precautions are taken. ●

While the possibility of becoming exposed to dangerous pathogens cannot be completely eliminated, there are many things you can do to minimize exposure. The first step is to understand that pathogens can live in nearly all types of body fluids, such as blood, vomit, urine, saliva, and tears. Minimizing exposure to all body fluids is key.

The term **standard precautions** is used to describe the set of infection-prevention practices health-care personnel use when caring for ill or injured people.[1] It includes the underlying philosophy that *all* ill or injured people (universally) should be considered potentially infectious and that you should take the necessary precautions to properly minimize exposure to body fluids.

3.4 Define the term *standard precautions* and how it relates to the Emergency Responder.

standard precautions the set of infection-prevention practices that health-care personnel use when caring for ill and injured people.

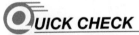

QUICK CHECK

Standard precautions are meant to protect you from exposure to potentially infectious blood and bodily fluids from which types of ill or injured people? ●

Taking Precautions

Our skin does an excellent job of keeping harmful pathogens from entering the body. However, the skin easily can be damaged by cuts and scrapes. These openings can allow germs access to the body.

Body substance isolation (BSI) precautions are precautions that an Emergency Responder must take to minimize exposure to blood and other potentially infectious material. BSI precautions include a variety of **personal protective equipment** that when used properly will minimize exposure to pathogens (▼ Figure 3.2). The following list includes some of the most common types of personal protective equipment:

- **Protective gloves.** These may be latex or non-latex and should be used at all times when caring for ill or injured people (Scan 3.1).

3.5 Define body substance isolation (BSI) precautions and when they should be used.

body substance isolation (BSI) precautions precautions taken to minimize exposure to blood and other potentially infectious material, typically through the use of protective gloves and eyewear.

personal protective equipment equipment, such as protective gloves and eyewear, that minimizes exposure to pathogens.

3.6 List examples of personal protective equipment and the purpose of each.

---

[1]The Occupational Safety and Health Administration (OSHA) Bloodborne Pathogen Standard 1910.1030 uses the term *universal precautions* as an approach to infection control. The U.S. Department of Health and Human Services (HHS) Centers for Disease Control and Prevention (CDC) guidelines combine the terms *universal precautions* and *body substance isolation* into a single set of precautions, *standard precautions*, for the care of patients in hospitals. Isolation practices and terminology continue to develop. For compliance with OSHA standards, the use of either universal precautions or standard precautions is acceptable.

Figure 3.2 The use of personal protective equipment will minimize exposure to dangerous pathogens.

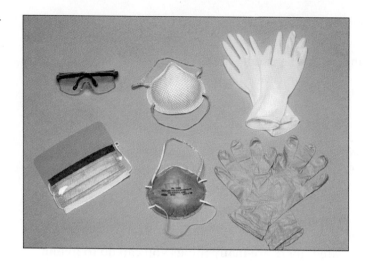

Proper Removal of Protective Gloves

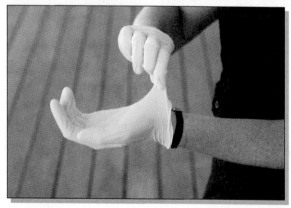

3.1.1 Begin by grasping the outer cuff of the opposite glove.

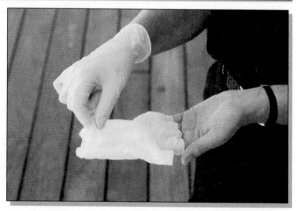

3.1.2 Carefully slip the glove over the hand, pulling it inside out.

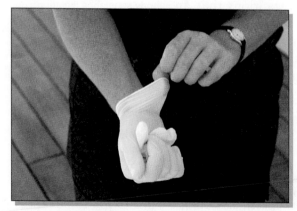

3.1.3 Next, slip a finger of the ungloved hand under the cuff.

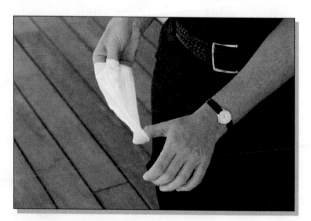

3.1.4 Carefully slip it off, turning it inside out.

Once removed, both gloves will end up inside out with one glove inside the other. This will contain any blood and body fluids.

- **Eye protection.** These may be in the form of safety goggles or a face shield, and their function is to protect the eyes from being splashed with fluids.
- **Masks.** These generally cover the nose and mouth and protect from splashed fluids as well as from inhaled pathogens.

Even the best attempts at minimizing exposure can fail. If you suffer a direct exposure to a person's blood or body fluids, you should immediately wash the area with soap and warm water.

3.7 Explain the procedure the Emergency Responder should follow after a possible exposure.

Every employer that has employees with a risk of occupational exposure to blood or other potentially infectious materials must perform an assessment of this risk and develop a written exposure-control plan intended to eliminate or minimize the risk. The plan must be accessible whenever an employee or the employee's designated representative requests it. Become familiar with your employer's written exposure-control plan. It will help guide you through the steps following an exposure. In most instances you will be evaluated by a physician, who will advise you on what steps you should take to minimize the chances of acquiring an illness due to the exposure.

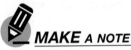

MAKE A NOTE

Just because you have been exposed does not mean you will become infected. By staying healthy and maintaining a strong immune system, and with proper post exposure measures, you can greatly minimize the chances of ever becoming infected. ●

Cleaning Up

Caring for ill or injured people is not the only time you could be at risk for exposure. Many times you will be at risk during the cleanup following an emergency. Naturally, you always will want to wash your hands thoroughly after assisting at an emergency. Your equipment must be cleaned and readied for the next response as well.

3.8 Differentiate between cleaning and disinfection, and state when each should be performed.

Proper cleanup is often a two-step process. You must first clean all equipment with warm, soapy water and then disinfect it with an appropriate disinfecting agent, such as isopropyl alcohol. It is important to understand that most disinfectants will not do a good job if the surfaces they are used on are dirty. That is why they must be free of any visible material, such as blood or vomit, to have the best chance of adequately disinfecting.

STRESSES OF BEING AN EMERGENCY RESPONDER

It is true. The responsibility of responding to emergency scenes and making decisions about what care an ill or injured person might require is stressful. In fact, it is often stressful for those who do it for a living. They just happen to enjoy that kind of stress.

3.9 Define the terms *stress* and *stressor* as they relate to the Emergency Responder.

The first step in developing good coping mechanisms is to understand what stress is. Depending on where you look and the context in which it

stressor any event or situation that places extraordinary demands on a person's mental and/or emotional resources.

stress tension, or a state of mental or emotional strain or suspense; the normal response to an abnormal situation or incident.

critical incident stress the stress that one experiences when faced with a significant event.

appears, there are many definitions of stress. The following are commonly accepted definitions:

- **Stressor.** A **stressor** is any event or situation that places extraordinary demands on a person's mental and/or emotional resources.
- **Stress.** **Stress** is tension, or a state of mental or emotional strain or suspense when one is exposed to stressors. It is the normal response to an abnormal situation or incident.

Sometimes the stress of responding to an emergency is lumped into a single definition called **critical incident stress**. A critical incident is any incident that causes someone to experience an extreme emotional response. Sometimes these reactions can affect one's ability to function normally.

Common Causes of Stress

3.10 Describe several sources of stressors commonly encountered by the Emergency Responder.

Emergency Responders deal with stress every day. A busy work schedule, aggressive deadlines, and challenging relationships are all stressors that you have become accustomed to dealing with and hopefully have learned to manage. Your decision to become trained in providing emergency care will indeed bring added stressors into your life. Knowing what to expect is the first step in your ability to properly manage them and develop appropriate coping mechanisms.

The expectation that you will know what to do and that you will respond appropriately during an emergency is one of the most common stressors for any Emergency Responder (▼ Figure 3.3). The possibility of seeing someone, especially someone you know, with a significant injury is another very common stressor.

The seriousness or horror of an incident is a factor in determining the amount of stress. Providing care for a seriously ill or injured child is generally more emotionally difficult than caring for an adult.

Add these stressors to the fact that your safety could be at risk when responding to an emergency scene and you have enough stress to be overwhelmed.

Common Responses to Stress

3.11 Describe common physical, emotional, and behavioral responses to stress.

Stress responses can vary widely. Some individuals may be immediately affected, while others may not begin to show signs of stress for some time. So how

Figure 3.3 Rescuers stand near the rubble of the fallen World Trade Center in New York, September 13, 2001. (© Reuters/CORBIS)

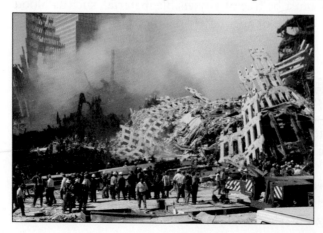

will you know if stress is beginning to affect you? The following is a list of some of the more common signs and symptoms of stress.

Physical Responses

- Fatigue
- Nausea/vomiting
- Difficulty sleeping
- Chest pain
- Rapid heart rate
- Difficulty concentrating
- Nightmares
- Difficulty making decisions

Emotional Responses

- Denial
- Fear
- Guilt
- Grief
- Anxiety
- Panic attacks
- Anger
- Depression

Behavioral Responses

- Withdrawal
- Inability to rest
- Antisocial behavior
- Increased use of alcohol
- Decreased appetite

Managing Stress

Most Emergency Responders want to believe that just about anything in life can be handled. In reality, stress affects everyone and can build up over time, resulting in a major crisis. Recognizing the signs and symptoms of stress can help you manage your own responses as well as offer assistance to those around you who may need a willing ear or shoulder to lean on.

3.12 Describe strategies for minimizing the affects of stress on the Emergency Responder.

The following is a list of simple ways that can help manage the stress in your life:

- Talk about what is bothering you.
- Eat a balanced diet.
- Get regular exercise. (▼ Figure 3.4)
- Make sure to schedule rest time in your day.
- Get plenty of sleep.

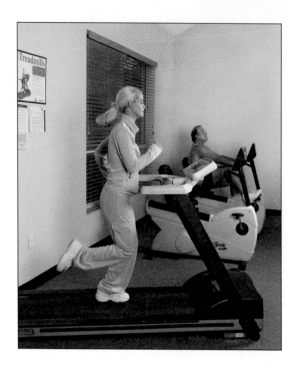

Figure 3.4 A healthy, balanced life includes regular exercise and a good diet.

Stress reactions are a normal human response to a traumatic event and are usually temporary. With the help of coworkers, family, and friends, most people gradually feel better as time goes by. If you feel you need extra help coping after a traumatic event, call your doctor. The organization you work for may have an employee assistance program available to assist you.

Our goal is not to scare you away from serving as an Emergency Responder. In fact, just the opposite is true. People become ill and injured every day, and most are cared for and comforted by Emergency Responders just like you. Our goal in sharing this information is to help keep you well informed and healthy, and to ensure you remain so as long as you choose to serve as an Emergency Responder.

THE HANDOFF

As your truck rumbles onto Burke Avenue, you see a mass of elementary school children all jostling for a better view of the two vehicles—a sedan and a pickup truck, twisted together and leaking multicolored fluids onto the pavement. The fire engine rolls to a stop in the street, air brakes hissing briefly, as you climb out and walk toward the vehicles, pulling on a pair of exam gloves as you go.

Your muscles are tense, and you can feel your heart thudding heavily in your chest as you circle the vehicles, looking for any safety hazards, expecting at any moment to come across a child battered and broken by an impact with one of these vehicles.

"What happened?" A man with blood dripping from his nose is sitting behind the wheel of the pickup truck. "Why am I here?"

Secure that there are no hazards and relieved to see only this one person in or around the vehicles, you approach the pickup truck, introduce yourself, and stabilize the man's head with your gloved hands. "You were in a collision, sir, but we are here to help."

As you are keeping the driver's head stable, Roger appears and begins sizing an extrication collar. "The other driver wasn't hurt," he says. "She's standing over on the sidewalk with the police. Apparently there was no child involved."

Relief pours over you, relaxing your stomach and slowing your heart rate as Roger places the cervical collar onto the driver. Roger's hands are shaking slightly, and when he sees that you notice, he sighs, "You know, I think I'm going to start jogging, too."

CHAPTER REVIEW

Chapter Summary

- Emergency scenes are often hazardous and pose many potential risks for the Emergency Responder, including traffic, fire, exposure to body fluids, and hazardous materials.

- Safety must always be your top priority. If it is not safe, do not enter the scene. Call 911 and wait for professionals to make the scene safe to enter.

- Disease-causing germs are called pathogens and can enter the body by way of any one of the following: ingestion, injection, absorption, or inhalation.

- Standard precautions refer to a set of infection-prevention practices that health-care personnel use when caring for ill and injured people. Standard precautions include the underlying philosophy that all ill or injured people must be considered infectious; therefore, you must wear proper personal protective equipment whenever you provide care.

- Body substance isolation (BSI) precautions are those precautions that must be taken to minimize exposure to blood or any other potentially infectious material.

- Examples of personal protective equipment include gloves, goggles, and facemasks.

- If you become exposed to a person's body fluids, you must immediately wash the area with warm, soapy water and contact your local physician for further guidance.

- There are two distinct steps when cleaning yourself or your equipment after use. You must first clean the surface with warm, soapy water to remove any visible contaminant. You will then apply a disinfecting agent to the surface to kill any remaining pathogens.

- Stress is a state of mental or emotional strain or suspense. Stress is the normal response to an abnormal situation or incident. Stressors are those factors or events that cause us to feel stress.

- There are many things that can make being an Emergency Responder stressful, including making emergency care decisions, working in a risky environment, and having to care for someone you know.

- Stress can manifest in many forms, including emotional, behavioral, and physical ways.

- The first step in managing stress is to know the signs and symptoms as well as to learn how you personally respond to stress.

Quick Quiz

1. Which one of the following ill or injured people presents to the Emergency Responder the greatest risk of exposure to blood?

   a. A person with difficulty breathing

   b. A person complaining of chest pain

   c. A person with an altered mental status

   d. A person with an open wound to the forehead

2. You arrive at the scene of an emergency in the parking lot at work. You find a car that has crashed into a power pole with two people inside who are crying in pain. The power pole is leaning over and looks like it may fall at any moment. What should you do first?

   a. Prevent others from entering the scene and call 911.

   b. Drag the victims from the vehicle and call 911.

   c. Instruct the victims to exit the vehicle.

   d. Call the utility company.

3. You are assisting an injured worker who was cut severely by a large shard of glass. While helping him, you kneel down on some broken glass that was covered with blood. The glass causes several small cuts on your knee. This type of exposure would be referred to as:

   a. inhalation.

   b. injection.

   c. absorption.

   d. ingestion.

4. Using personal protective equipment such as gloves to protect yourself from being exposed to blood is also known as _____ precautions.

   a. work-related

   b. pathogen

   c. body substance isolation

   d. immediate

5. You have just finished helping at the scene of an emergency and notice some blood from the person on the back of your forearm. What should you do first?

   a. Immediately wash with soap and water.

   b. Follow the ambulance to the hospital.

   c. Notify your supervisor.

   d. Wipe it off with a dry towel.

6. Denial, fear, and guilt are signs and symptoms of what type of stress response?

   a. Physical

   b. Emotional

   c. Behavioral

   d. Psychological

7. You notice a coworker has become increasingly quiet and isolated following the death of another coworker earlier in the week. Which one of the following would be a good initial strategy for helping this person?

   a. Refer him to professional counseling.

   b. Demand that he tell you what is wrong.

   c. Ignore him. He must work through things alone.

   d. Encourage him to talk about the incident.

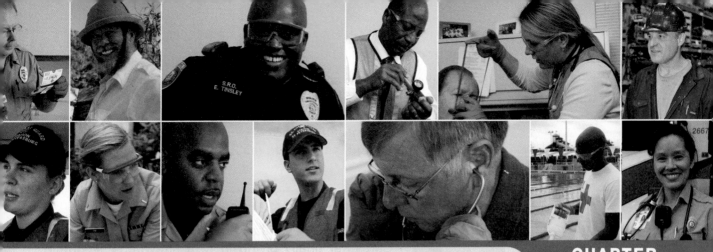

Introduction to Anatomy

LEARNING OBJECTIVES

At the conclusion of this chapter and the associated instructor-guided lesson, the student will be able to:

Cognitive

4.1 Describe the standard anatomical position. *(p. 36)*

4.2 Identify the four major body cavities. *(p. 38)*

4.3 Describe the anatomy and function of the respiratory system. *(p. 39)*

4.4 Describe the anatomy and function of the circulatory system. *(p. 40)*

4.5 Describe the anatomy and function of the musculoskeletal system. *(p. 42)*

4.6 Describe the anatomy and function of the nervous system. *(p. 44)*

4.7 Describe the anatomy and function of the skin. *(p. 45)*

KEY TERMS

The following terms are introduced in this chapter:

- anterior *(p. 37)*
- distal *(p. 38)*
- inferior *(p. 38)*
- lateral *(p. 37)*
- medial *(p. 37)*
- midline *(p. 37)*
- posterior *(p. 37)*
- prone *(p. 36)*
- proximal *(p. 37)*
- superior *(p. 38)*
- supine *(p. 36)*

Introduction

THIS chapter introduces some of the basic principles of human anatomy. While it is not essential that you fully understand how the body works and the relationship of one system to another, it can be very helpful when performing your assessment and when providing a description of the ill or injured person's signs and symptoms to the EMS team.

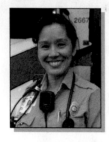

THE EMERGENCY

You are standing at the counter of the 42nd Street Juice Cart after finally giving in to a strawberry smoothie craving that has been following you for much of your shift. It started when a group of high school kids walked past you with the colorful, frosty drinks in their hands, slurping from thick straws as you were writing a ticket for a double-parked produce truck on Ninth Avenue.

"Here you go, officer." The woman running the cart hands you a large, cold cup and waves her hand when you hold up cash. "No charge. That one is on the house."

"That's kind of you," you say, dropping the cost of the smoothie into the tip jar anyway.

As you are turning from the counter to continue on your foot beat, an alarm starts clanging wildly half a block up the avenue. You hear several loud pops and see a man in a scruffy blue jacket carrying a small silver handgun and crashing through the door from Benny's Pawn Shop. He stumbles down the stairs, eyes darting around wildly, and runs off toward the docks. You set your drink back on the cart's Formica counter, relay the incident and the man's description to dispatch over your radio, and run the half block to Benny's.

With heart racing, you enter the small, cluttered shop with your weapon drawn. You are met by the stinging scent of gunpowder and low moans from behind a smashed jewelry display case. You move carefully across the shop and peer around the end of the counter. You see Benny's grandson, who sometimes works in the shop when home from college, lying in a pool of blood on the worn linoleum floor.

4.1 Describe the standard anatomical position.

supine lying face up.

prone lying facedown.

ANATOMICAL POSITION

There is no telling what position you might find an injured or ill person in. Such a person could be face up (**supine**), facedown (**prone**), on his side (lateral), or in any one of a dozen other awkward positions. Without a standard reference point, attempting to describe where there is pain or where an injury is located could be difficult. For this reason, health-care providers use something called the anatomical position.

The **anatomical position** is the position that is assumed whenever the body or its parts are described. It is achieved with a person standing upright

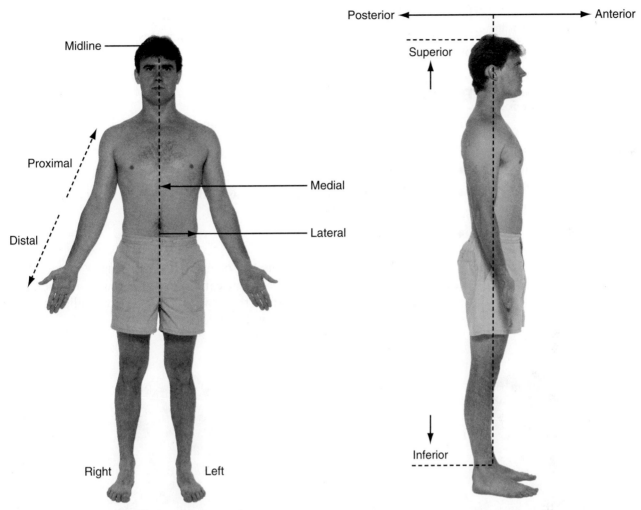

Figure 4.1 Anatomical position and directional terms.

with arms extended down at the sides and the palms of the hands facing forward. ▲ Figure 4.1 shows a person in the anatomical position. The illustration also includes some of the more common directional terms:

- **Anterior.** The front of the body
- **Posterior.** The back of the body
- **Medial.** Toward the midline of the body
- **Lateral.** Toward the side of the body
- **Midline.** The middle of the body
- **Proximal.** Closer to the torso (in reference to a limb)
- **Distal.** Further from the torso (in reference to a limb)
- **Inferior.** Toward the feet
- **Superior.** Toward the head

It is important to understand that when you say "left" and "right" to describe an ill or injured person's condition (e.g., "She is complaining of pain

anterior the front of the body; e.g., the navel (belly button) is located on the anterior abdomen.

posterior the back of the body; e.g., the shoulder blades are located on the posterior side of the torso.

medial toward the midline of the body; e.g., the pinky is located on the medial side of the hand.

lateral toward the side of the body; e.g., the thumb is on the lateral side of the hand.

midline the center of the body; e.g., the navel is located on the abdomen directly on the midline.

proximal closer to the torso (in reference to a limb); e.g., the shoulder is proximal to the elbow.

distal further from the torso (in reference to a limb); e.g., the hand is distal to the elbow.

inferior toward the feet; e.g., the chin is inferior to the mouth.

superior toward the head; e.g., the nose is superior to the mouth.

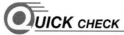UICK CHECK

Describe a person who is in the anatomical position. ●

4.2 Identify the four major body cavities.

in her left shoulder"), it is assumed that you are referring to the ill or injured person's left or right, not that of the Emergency Responder. Always refer only to the ill or injured person's left or right.

BODY CAVITIES

There are four main cavities within the human body:

- Head (brain)
- Chest (heart and lungs)
- Abdomen (liver, intestines, pancreas, kidneys, spleen, stomach, and gall bladder)
- Pelvis (intestines and bladder)

Each of these cavities contains one or more body organs (▼ Figure 4.2). With the exception of the head, each one can hide enough internal blood loss to be life threatening. It is important to know this and be extra diligent when assessing an injured or ill person with pain in these areas.

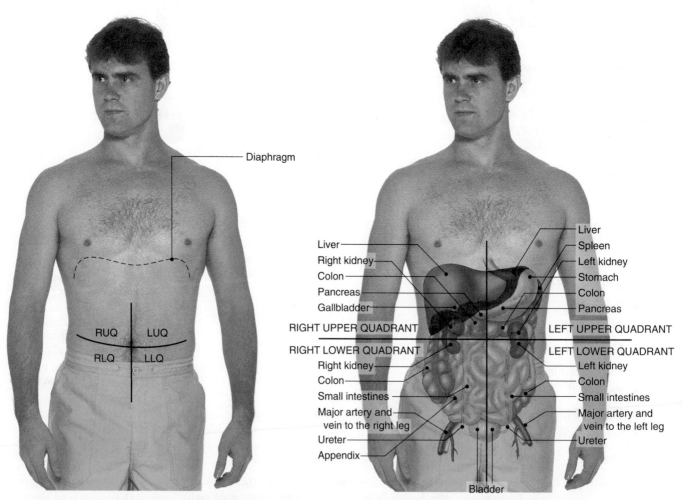

Figure 4.2 The quadrants of the abdomen and the organs located in each.

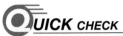
Which of the four main body cavities can hide enough blood loss to be life threatening? ●

RESPIRATORY SYSTEM

The respiratory system is made up of the nose, mouth, trachea, and lungs (▼ Figure 4.3). It is responsible for the intake of fresh oxygen and the removal of waste in the form of carbon dioxide. The air we breathe is

4.3 Describe the anatomy and function of the respiratory system.

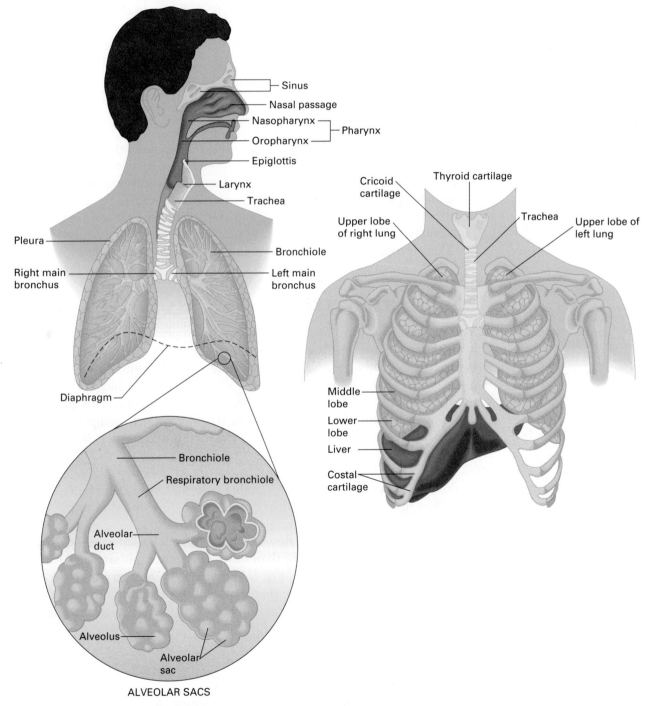

Figure 4.3 The respiratory system.

approximately 21 percent oxygen, which enters the body through the nose and mouth each time we take in a breath (inhale). The air travels down the windpipe (trachea) and eventually enters the lungs. Deep inside the lungs, the oxygen is able to enter the bloodstream and eventually be carried throughout the body, where it is used as fuel for the cells. Without a constant supply of oxygen, the cells of the body will die. When enough cells die, the entire body dies.

Bringing oxygen into the body is really only half the story. It is just as important that the respiratory system remove waste in the form of carbon dioxide to maintain a healthy state of being. Each time we breathe out (exhale) the body removes carbon dioxide and rids the body of this waste material.

 PEDIATRIC CARE

One of the biggest differences between adults and children is the size of the airway. Due to the small size of a child's airway, it is much more prone to obstruction. ●

Maintaining a constant and steady exchange of oxygen and carbon dioxide is the main purpose of the respiratory system. It does this by adjusting the number of times we breathe (rate) and the amount of air we take in with each breath (volume).

The appropriate method for assessing breathing is discussed in Chapter 6.

CIRCULATORY SYSTEM

4.4 Describe the anatomy and function of the circulatory system.

Much like oxygen, the body needs a steady supply of blood to the cells to keep all the organs and body systems functioning properly. The circulatory system is made up of the heart, blood vessels, and the blood (▶ Figure 4.4). Used blood from the body enters the right side of the heart and is then pumped out to the lungs, where it becomes oxygenated. This now fresh blood flows back to the left side of the heart, where it gets pumped out to the body. The cycle begins all over again as the used blood reenters the right side of the heart.

There are many things that can disrupt the circulatory system or one of its three components. Heart attack, damage to the vessels, and blood loss all can affect the circulatory system and reduce the flow of blood to the body's vital organs.

Blood that is oxygenated flows through vessels called arteries. Arteries are under much higher pressure than other vessels and pulsate each time the heart beats. The other vessels are called veins. Veins carry deoxygenated blood back to the heart and are under much less pressure than arteries. For this reason, blood coming from an injured vein is often darker red in color and flows steadily from the wound.

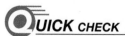 **QUICK** CHECK

Blood traveling from the right side of the heart goes where? ●

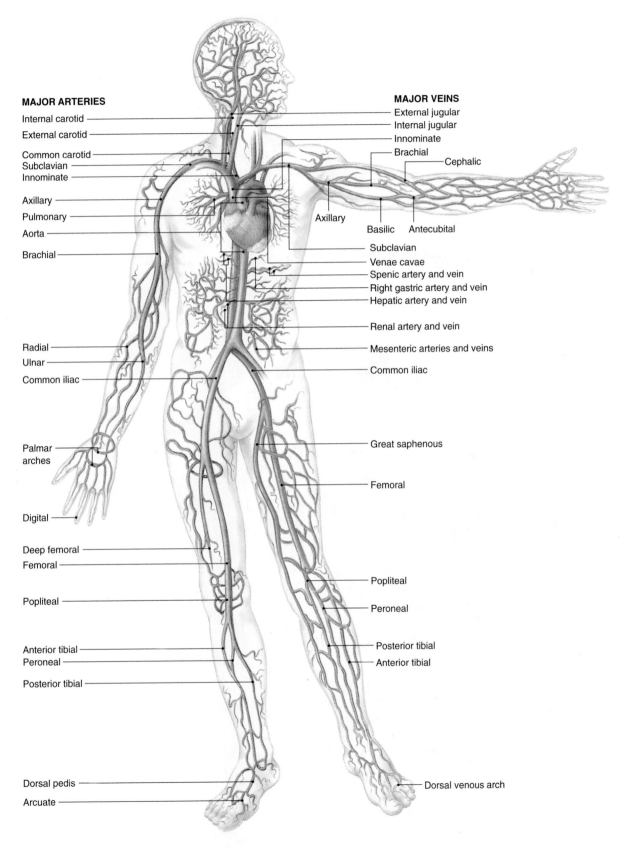

MAJOR ARTERIES

Internal carotid
External carotid
Common carotid
Subclavian
Innominate
Axillary
Pulmonary
Aorta
Brachial
Radial
Ulnar
Common iliac
Palmar arches
Digital
Deep femoral
Femoral
Popliteal
Anterior tibial
Peroneal
Posterior tibial
Dorsal pedis
Arcuate

MAJOR VEINS

External jugular
Internal jugular
Innominate
Brachial
Cephalic
Axillary
Basilic
Antecubital
Subclavian
Venae cavae
Spenic artery and vein
Right gastric artery and vein
Hepatic artery and vein
Renal artery and vein
Mesenteric arteries and veins
Common iliac
Great saphenous
Femoral
Popliteal
Peroneal
Posterior tibial
Anterior tibial
Dorsal venous arch

Figure 4.4 The circulatory system.

MUSCULOSKELETAL SYSTEM

4.5 Describe the anatomy and function of the musculoskeletal system.

The musculoskeletal system is made up of muscles and bones, which together give us our shape and ability to move about (▼ Figure 4.5). The skeletal system provides several functions, such as movement, protection of vital organs, and blood cell production. While bones are not typically thought of as a vital system, injuries to bones can be very painful.

Bones can suffer injuries such as cracks, breaks, and bruises. It is often difficult to determine what type of muscle or bone injury the person has. For this reason, you will most often care for any painful musculoskeletal injury as if there is a broken bone.

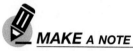 **MAKE** *A* *NOTE*

While they can be very painful, isolated injuries to muscles and bones are rarely life threatening. The focus of your care for people with musculoskeletal injuries will be on keeping them still to help minimize pain. ●

Figure 4.5a The musculoskeletal system: skeleton.

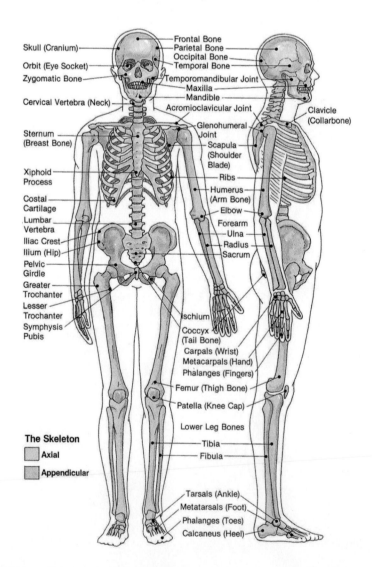

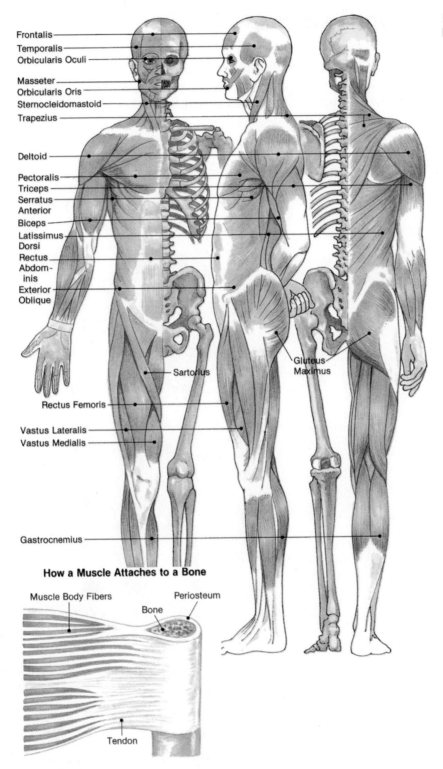

Figure 4.5b The musculoskeletal system: muscles.

Frontalis
Temporalis
Orbicularis Oculi

Masseter
Orbicularis Oris
Sternocleidomastoid
Trapezius

Deltoid

Pectoralis
Triceps
Serratus Anterior
Biceps
Latissimus Dorsi
Rectus Abdominis
Exterior Oblique

Sartorius

Gluteus Maximus

Rectus Femoris

Vastus Lateralis
Vastus Medialis

Gastrocnemius

How a Muscle Attaches to a Bone

Muscle Body Fibers
Periosteum
Bone
Tendon

Much like the bones, the muscles have several functions, such as movement, protection, and heat production. Muscles also can suffer injuries that are very painful. The two main types of injury to a muscle are strains and tears. These most often occur when a muscle is overworked or overextended. The care for injuries to the muscles and bones will be discussed in Chapter 10.

NERVOUS SYSTEM

4.6 Describe the anatomy and function of the nervous system.

The nervous system is made up of the brain, spinal cord, and nerves (▼ Figure 4.6). It is the brain that controls most of the body's functions, and it does so by sending and receiving messages through the spinal cord and nerve endings. The nervous system is further divided into the central

Figure 4.6 The nervous system.

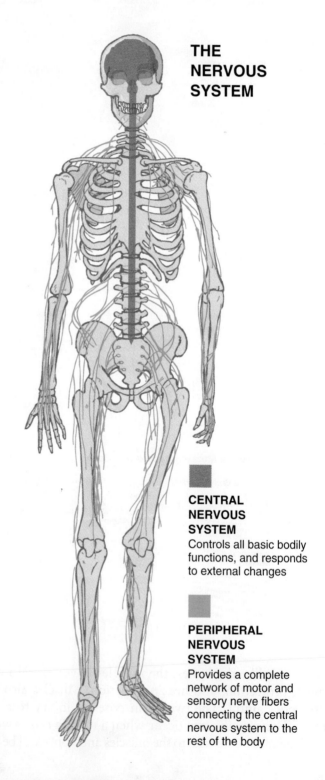

THE
NERVOUS
SYSTEM

CENTRAL NERVOUS SYSTEM
Controls all basic bodily functions, and responds to external changes

PERIPHERAL NERVOUS SYSTEM
Provides a complete network of motor and sensory nerve fibers connecting the central nervous system to the rest of the body

nervous system, which includes the brain and spinal cord, and the peripheral nervous system, which includes all the nerves that extend from the spinal cord.

THE SKIN

So often we take our skin for granted. Rarely does anyone think of the skin as a separate organ system, but it is. The skin covers nearly every square inch of the body and serves many important functions. It performs those functions with little awareness by us, unless, of course, it becomes damaged or fails in some way.

4.7 Describe the anatomy and function of the skin.

First and foremost, our skin is an amazingly effective first line of defense against infection from pathogens. It also helps to protect us from our environment by regulating body temperature. It is the skin that contains the millions of tiny nerve endings that allow us to sense touch, pain, pressure, and heat and cold.

The skin is made up of three layers (▼ Figure 4.7):

- **Epidermis.** This is the outermost layer of skin.
- **Dermis.** This layer lies beneath the epidermis and contains the sweat and oil glands, hair follicles, nerve endings, and some blood vessels.
- **Subcutaneous.** This is the deepest layer of skin and is made up of fatty tissue, which provides shock absorption and insulation for the body.

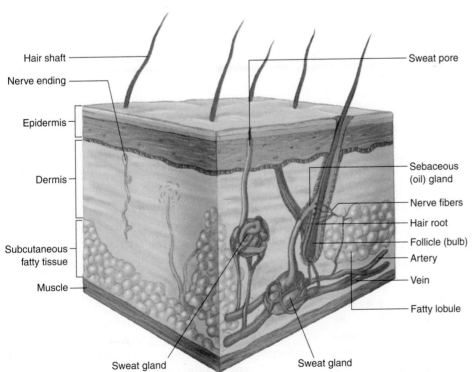

Figure 4.7 The layers of the skin.

Hair shaft
Nerve ending
Epidermis
Dermis
Subcutaneous fatty tissue
Muscle
Sweat gland
Sweat gland
Sweat pore
Sebaceous (oil) gland
Nerve fibers
Hair root
Follicle (bulb)
Artery
Vein
Fatty lobule

THE HANDOFF

"Hang in there, Tim! I've already called for an ambulance." You quickly grab a pair of exam gloves from a pouch on your duty belt, and, after confirming that he is breathing and still conscious, you pull his shirt open. There are several holes punched through the pale skin of his chest and abdomen, and blood is running steadily from one of them.

You apply pressure to the bleeding hole with one gloved hand and key your portable with the other. "Central, seven-frank-nineteen."

"Frank-nineteen, go ahead."

"Central, I need you to relay info to the responding medical crew. The person is breathing, but it seems shallow and pained. I count three gunshot wounds, all entrance wounds and in the anterior torso. Two are in the chest, just superior to the right nipple, and one is right on the midline, inferior to the navel. I checked the posterior and found no obvious exit wounds."

"Copy that, frank-nineteen. We're passing it along now."

After what seems like much longer than it actually is, an ambulance crew comes through the door, hauling equipment boxes and an airway bag to the young man's side. After checking in with the person and ensuring that her partner was preparing the oxygen, the paramedic kneels next to you on the old floor.

"Great job on the report," she says, placing a dressing over the bleeding wound so you can move your gloved hand. "It really gave us an idea of what to anticipate. I wish I went into every call with that kind of detail!"

CHAPTER REVIEW

Chapter Summary

- For purposes of standardization and consistency, it is appropriate to describe signs, symptoms, and injuries of an injured or ill person as if he or she were in the anatomical position. The anatomical position is one in which the person is standing upright, facing forward with arms extended down at the side with the palms facing forward.

- The four major body cavities are the head, chest, abdomen, and pelvis. Each of these areas contains major organs, and all but the head can hide internal blood loss.

- The respiratory system is made up of the mouth, nose, trachea, and lungs and is responsible for the intake of fresh oxygen from the air and the elimination of wastes in the form of carbon dioxide. The respiratory system is regulated by the brain and adjusts rate (how fast) and volume (how much) of our breaths depending on the body's needs.

- The circulatory system is made up of the heart, vessels, and blood and is responsible for the circulation of blood to all cells of the body.

- The musculoskeletal system is made up of the muscles and bones and is the system that provides us with our basic shape and ability to move.

- The nervous system is made up of the brain, spinal cord, and nerves. It is this system that controls all voluntary and involuntary actions of the body.

- The skin is made up of the dermis, epidermis, and subcutaneous layers. It is vital for temperature regulation as well as great protection against pathogens and the environment.

Quick Quiz

1. An advantage to using the anatomical position when describing the location of an injury is that:

   a. it allows for easy identification of wound types.

   b. the person will understand what is wrong with her.

   c. others will understand what you are describing.

   d. it is the only legal way to describe an injury.

2. Which body cavity contains the liver, spleen, and much of the large intestine?

   a. Skull

   b. Chest

   c. Abdomen

   d. Pelvis

3. The brain controls the respirations by adjusting breathing rate and:

   a. volume.

   b. regularity.

   c. strength.

   d. temperature.

4. The heart, vessels, and blood are all components of which body system?

   a. Respiratory

   b. Circulatory

   c. Musculoskeletal

   d. Nervous

5. Which body system is divided into two subsystems—the central and peripheral systems?

   a. Respiratory

   b. Circulatory

   c. Musculoskeletal

   d. Nervous

6. All of the following are functions of the musculoskeletal system EXCEPT:

   a. support.

   b. movement.

   c. temperature regulation.

   d. protection.

7. Which layer of the skin is the outermost layer and provides the protection against the environment and pathogens?

   a. Dermis

   b. Epidermis

   c. Subcutaneous

   d. Sebaceous

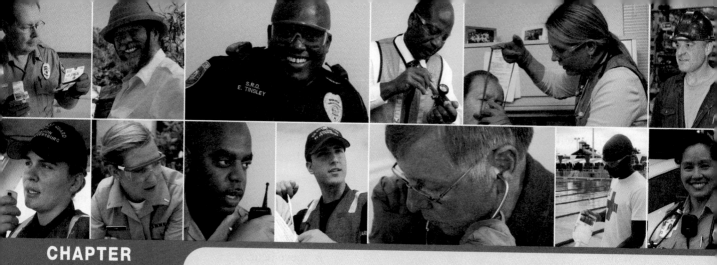

Principles of Lifting, Moving, and Positioning

KEY TERMS

The following terms are introduced in this chapter:

- body mechanics *(p. 49)*
- chair lift *(p. 56)*
- clothes drag *(p. 57)*
- emergent move *(p. 50)*
- extremity lift *(p. 55)*
- log roll *(p. 54)*
- recovery position *(p. 53)*
- stair chair *(p. 56)*

LEARNING OBJECTIVES

At the conclusion of this chapter and the associated instructor-guided lesson, the student will be able to:

Cognitive

5.1 Explain when it would be necessary to move an injured or ill person. *(p. 49)*

5.2 Explain the importance of using proper body mechanics. *(p. 51)*

5.3 Describe the characteristics of proper body mechanics. *(p. 52)*

5.4 Explain the risks of not using proper body mechanics when lifting and moving an ill or injured person. *(p. 51)*

5.5 Explain the importance of active communication during lifts and moves. *(p. 52)*

5.6 Explain the purpose of the recovery position, and state when it should be used. *(p. 53)*

5.7 Describe the common techniques used for moving ill or injured people. *(p. 52)*

Psychomotor

5.8 Demonstrate the use of proper body mechanics while performing ill or injured person moves.

5.9 Demonstrate the proper technique for log rolling an ill or injured person.

5.10 Demonstrate the proper technique for placing a supine ill or injured person into the recovery position.

5.11 Demonstrate the proper technique for performing a log roll, extremity lift, stair chair or chair lift, and a clothes drag.

Introduction

THERE may be times when it will be necessary to move an ill or injured person. There are many things that make moving ill or injured people risky, not the least of which is possible injury to you or others assisting you. This chapter addresses when and when not to move someone and the potential risks to both you and the person you are moving. It also describes proper **body mechanics** and a variety of techniques that you can use to move someone safely.

body mechanics refers to the proper use of the body to facilitate moving and lifting with the goal of maximizing effectiveness and minimizing personal injury.

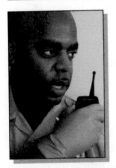

THE EMERGENCY

The downtown mall is deserted except for a single shopper slowly wandering between storefronts, peering disinterestedly into each window for a moment before moving on. The sound of his footfalls and the crinkle of a single plastic bag hanging limply at the end of his arm echoes through the bright, cavernous shopping plaza.

"Go check the parking structure," Randy, the mall security shift supervisor, says to you as you both lean against the mezzanine railing, waiting out the last few minutes before the mall closes. "That guy's car will be the only thing out there."

You smile and nod toward the lone shopper now at the far end of the mall, his face against a window. When Randy doesn't smile back, you push off and walk toward the large glass doors leading to the parking area.

The evening air is cool and smells like rain, and you are looking at the clouds building in the sky when you hear the loud, shuddering squeal of tires followed by a crash. You jog to the end of the building and turn the corner, nervous about what you are about to find.

Debris is scattered across the road, and you see a badly damaged car half up on the curb, hood open, with dark smoke billowing from the engine compartment. You contact Randy on the portable radio and tell him to activate EMS.

"Help me!" You hear someone yell, but you don't see a driver in the car. "Please somebody help!"

You circle the smoking car from a distance and see a man lying on the ground near the open driver's door. He is bleeding profusely from a head wound, and when he sees you he reaches one arm out and continues yelling for help. As you start to approach him, you notice quickly growing flames now pushing through the smoke from the engine compartment.

MAKING THE DECISION TO MOVE

In most situations it is best to leave the ill or injured person in the position that you find him. In fact, most of the time the person has found a position that is most comfortable for his condition and the pain that he is experiencing. This is not to say that he is not in pain. It only means that he has probably found a position that offers the least amount of pain for his illness or injury.

5.1 Explain when it would be necessary to move an injured or ill person.

Simply stated, do not be in a big hurry to move someone until you have had a chance to evaluate the situation and the person's condition.

EMERGENT VS. NONEMERGENT MOVES

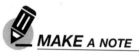

emergent move a move that is necessary when there is an immediate threat to an ill or injured person's life.

There are specific conditions for which it may be necessary to move an ill or injured person and move him quickly. This type of move is often referred to as an **emergent move**. You would use an emergent move because of an immediate external threat to the ill or injured person (▼ Figure 5.1). For example, consider a woman who has been injured by a piece of falling debris. There is an immediate danger that she could be struck again by more falling debris. You would want to move her to a safer location to prevent further injury. Now please remember that you must keep your personal safety in mind at all times and not expose yourself to undue risk. If it is not safe to approach an injured or ill person, do not do so. Call 911 and wait for trained professionals to arrive and assist.

Another reason you may need to use an emergent move involves a person who is experiencing an immediate problem related to the airway, breathing, circulation, or severe bleeding. If not addressed immediately, any one of those conditions could result in death for the ill or injured person. You must carefully and quickly move the person into a position that will allow you to properly provide care. For example, imagine you have been called to an injured man who has fallen from a height and is lying facedown on the ground. A quick assessment reveals that he is not breathing. You must carefully and quickly roll this person onto his back so you can properly open the airway and provide rescue breaths as necessary. If not, the person is certainly going to die.

MAKE A NOTE

You will never be expected to put yourself at undue risk to help another person. While Emergency Responders are exposed to risks and hazards all the time, you must carefully consider the risks and do what you can to minimize harm to yourself and others before attempting to render aid to an injured or ill person. ●

Figure 5.1 An emergent move is one that must be made quickly because of an immediate threat to the ill or injured person.

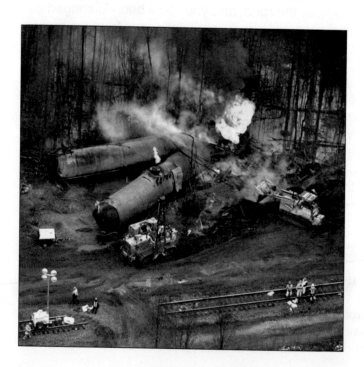

So you see, there are certain times when moving an ill or injured person is the right thing to do, even before you complete a thorough assessment. These situations are relatively uncommon, but you must be ready when they arise.

For the most part, the moves that you use will likely be nonemergent and help facilitate a more thorough assessment.

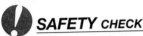

SAFETY CHECK

One of the most important safety concerns when considering moving or lifting an ill or injured person is whether you have enough people to assist you. The number of people you will need will depend on the size of the ill or injured person and the size of your helpers. Never attempt to lift or move an ill or injured person if you do not have adequate help. ●

PROPER BODY MECHANICS

To minimize risk of injury to yourself and anyone who may be assisting you while moving an ill or injured person, you must understand and utilize proper body mechanics. Good body mechanics involve the proper use of your body to facilitate moving and lifting with the goal of maximizing effectiveness and minimizing personal injury.

5.2 Explain the importance of using proper body mechanics.

Lifting and moving improperly can result in anything from a simple pulled muscle to a severely injured back. Injuries to the trunk, including the shoulder and back, account for more than 30 percent of all occupational injuries.[1] Not taking the time to size up the situation, to ensure that you have enough assistance, and to use good body mechanics can easily result in significant injury to you and anyone assisting you with moving (▼ Figure 5.2). There is already one ill or injured person. Do not add yourself or those assisting you to that list.

5.4 Explain the risks of not using proper body mechanics when lifting and moving an ill or injured person.

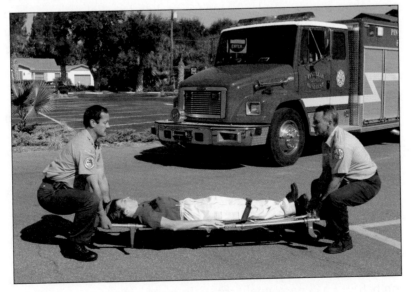

Figure 5.2 Plan how you will perform a lift, be sure you have enough assistance, and always use proper body mechanics.

[1]U.S. Bureau of Labor Statistics, *Nonfatal Occupational Injuries and Illnesses Requiring Days away from Work*, 2008. USDL-09-1454 (Washington, DC: U.S. Bureau of Labor Statistics, 2009), http://www.bls.gov/news.release/osh2.nr0.htm (accessed January 11, 2010).

Most people get by day in and day out without using good body mechanics. Since most are not typically moving or lifting heavy objects, they can easily compensate and never become injured. You may be required to move an ill or injured person and must use good body mechanics to do it as safely as possible. It is important to understand that at first good body mechanics will feel awkward and clumsy, especially if you have already developed poor habits. Any time you are attempting to make a change to improve body mechanics, it will feel awkward, but the more you practice them, the sooner you will feel comfortable and the sooner you will make the improved motion a natural thing to do.

The following is a list of key concepts related to good body mechanics. Learn these concepts and make a strong effort to practice them each day:

- **Position your feet properly.** They should be on a firm, level surface and positioned a comfortable width apart. Take extra care if the surface is slippery or unstable.

- **Lift with your legs.** Keep your back as straight as possible and bend at your knees. Try not to bend at the waist any more than you absolutely have to.

- **Avoid leaning to either side.** When lifting with one hand, bend your knees to grasp the object, and keep your back straight.

- **Minimize twisting during a lift.** Attempts to turn or twist while you are lifting can result in serious injury.

- **Keep the weight as close to your body as possible.** The farther the weight is from your body, the greater your chance of injury.

THE IMPORTANCE OF GOOD COMMUNICATION

One of the most important elements of a successful lift or move that involves more than one responder is good visual and verbal communication. One of the easiest ways to cause an injury is for one responder to lift or move before the other responders are ready. To avoid these types of mistakes you must ensure that someone is assigned to coordinate the move verbally and that all responders are making eye contact before the move is initiated.

Typically, the person at the head of the ill or injured person will initiate the lift or move once he has ensured that all other responders are aware of the plan and are ready to go. Using a simple 1-2-3 count, he can coordinate the move so that everyone moves at the same time and keeps the ill or injured person as stable as possible.

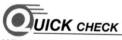

QUICK **CHECK**

Which is the best way to avoid injury—holding a heavy object close to or far from your body? ●

COMMON MOVES

The following text will introduce a few of the most common techniques you can use to move an ill or injured person when it becomes necessary. Remember, your job is to comfort, assess, and stabilize an ill or injured person before EMS personnel arrives. In most instances you will not be required to lift or move the ill or injured person. The following moves and lifts can all be used for emergent or nonemergent situations, depending on the person's condition and the hazards of the environment.

Recovery Position

One of the most important moves you will need to know is how to correctly place an ill or injured person into what is called the **recovery position**. The recovery position is used for responsive or unresponsive people who are found lying down with adequate breathing and circulation and whom you do not suspect have a neck or spinal injury. It involves placing the person onto her side to assist with keeping the airway clear and minimize the chances of choking, should she vomit. The following steps should be followed when placing an ill or injured person in the recovery position (Scan 5.1):

1. Kneel beside the ill or injured person on her left side. Raise her left arm straight out above her head.
2. Cross the person's right arm over her chest, placing her right hand next to her left cheek.
3. Raise the right knee until it is completely flexed.

5.6 Explain the purpose of the recovery position, and state when it should be used.

recovery position lying on the left side; a position that engages gravity to help keep the ill or injured person's airway clear.

SCAN 5.1   The Recovery Position

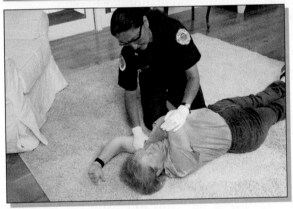

5.1.1 With the left arm raised above the head, cross the right arm over the chest, placing the right hand next to her left cheek.

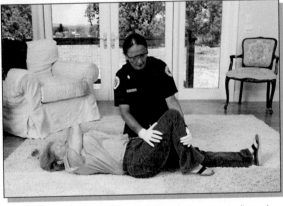

5.1.2 Raise the right knee until it is completely flexed.

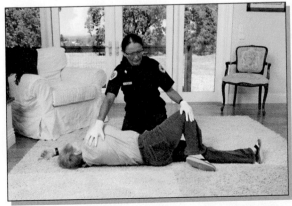

5.1.3 Using the knee and shoulder, carefully pull her onto her side.

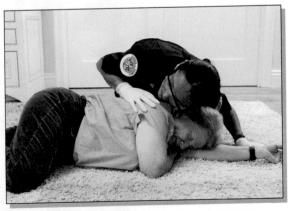

5.1.4 Adjust the knee and shoulder to stabilize her. Then recheck the airway, breathing, and circulation.

4. Place your right hand on the person's right shoulder and your left hand on her flexed right knee. Using the flexed knee as a lever, pull her toward you, guiding her torso in a smooth rolling motion onto her side. The person's head will rest on her left arm.

5. As best as you can, position her right elbow and knee on the floor so that they act like a kickstand, preventing the person from rolling completely onto her stomach. Place her right hand under the side of her face. The arm will support her in this position. The hand will cushion her face and allow the head to angle slightly downward for airway drainage.

Depending on the position in which the ill or injured person is found, you may place her on either her right or left side.

Log Roll

The **log roll** can be either an emergent or a nonemergent move, depending on the reason it is being used. It may be used to roll an ill or injured person from his back to his side should you need to clear the airway, control bleeding from the back, or place him onto a backboard. It also can be used to roll a person from a facedown position to a face-up position. This may be necessary if you discover problems with the airway, breathing, circulation, or bleeding.

One responder can perform a log roll, but the ideal number is three. With three, one can manage the head, keeping it in proper alignment with the spine, while the other two manage the rest of the body. The following steps should be followed when performing a three-person log roll (▼ Figure 5.3):

1. One responder should kneel at the top of the ill or injured person's head and hold or stabilize the head and neck in the position in which it was found. Notice which way the person's head is facing, because you will most likely want to roll in the opposite direction.

2. A second responder should kneel at the person's side opposite the direction the head is facing. Quickly assess the arms to ensure there are no

Figure 5.3 A three-rescuer log roll.

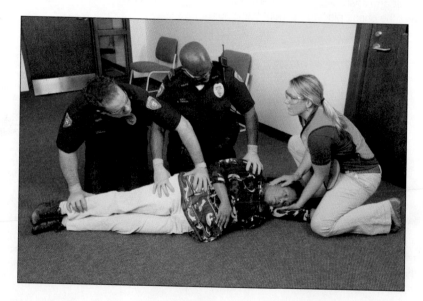

obvious injuries. Raise and extend the person's arm that is opposite the direction the head is facing. Position that arm straight up above the head. This allows for easy rolling to the side and provides support for the head during the roll. This is especially helpful if you must do the log roll alone.

3. The third responder should kneel at the person's hips.

4. Responders should grasp the person's shoulders, hips, knees, and ankles. If only one responder is available to roll the person, he should grasp the heavy parts of the torso (shoulders and hips).

5. The responder at the person's head should signal and give directions: "On three, slowly roll. One, two, three—roll together." All responders should slowly roll the person in a coordinated move and carefully keep the spine in a neutral, in-line position until the person is supine (face up).

It is important to note that the responder holding the head should not initially try to turn the head with the body. Since the head is already facing sideways, allow the body to come into alignment with the head. Once the body and head are aligned, approximately halfway through the roll, the responder at the head should then move with the body, keeping the head and body aligned until the person is in the supine position.

Extremity Lift

There may be times when an ill or injured person ends up on the ground and needs to be lifted to a chair, couch, or some type of stretcher. When it is clear that the person does not have a suspected neck or back injury, the **extremity lift** is ideal for this type of move. Follow these steps to perform an extremity lift (▼ Figure 5.4):

extremity lift a technique for moving an ill or injured person who is on the ground and must be lifted onto a chair or stretcher.

1. One responder should kneel behind the person and reach around with both hands to grasp the outside of the person's wrists. An alternate method is to reach around all the way and grasp the opposite wrist.

2. The second responder should kneel beside the person's knees and wrap both arms under them. It may be helpful to bring the person's knees into the bent position before attempting to place your arms underneath.

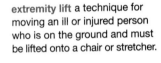

QUICK CHECK

For which ill or injured person is the extremity lift ideally suited? ●

3. At the direction of the responder at the head, both responders should stand up at the same time.

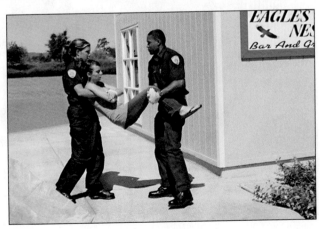

Figure 5.4 An extremity lift.

Stair Chair

Any organization where a sizable number of people work or gather should have an emergency plan, including an evacuation plan. The emergency plan should include procedures for evacuating physically handicapped, ill, or injured employees, visitors, or tenants during natural or other types of disasters when EMS personnel may be significantly delayed or even unavailable. While a variety of evacuation methods and products are available, the **stair chair** is the most common type of assistive device (▼ Figure 5.5).

There are several different stair chair options that vary in operation. All Emergency Responders should be familiar with the evacuation equipment available in their facility.

Where available, use of the stair chair should be incorporated into the facility evaluation plan, Emergency Responder training, and drills. Follow the manufacturer's instructions for proper use. The stair chair is NOT for someone who you suspect may have a neck or back injury.

Chair Lift

The **chair lift** is an alternative technique for moving an ill or injured person down stairs or out of a building when a stair chair is unavailable. Like the stair chair, the chair lift is NOT for someone who you suspect may have a neck or back injury.

To perform a chair lift, you must first select a household chair. It must be strong and sturdy and should preferably have arms. Then follow these steps:

1. Use the extremity lift to bring the person from the ground or floor to the chair.

2. One responder then should stand behind the chair and grab on securely to the back of the chair.

---

stair chair a device specifically designed to allow responders to move an ill or injured person down stairs safely.

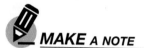

MAKE A NOTE

Some corporate or industrial settings have devices similar to the stair chair specifically designed for the evacuation of ill or injured people in the event of an emergency. You should be familiar with such devices and how to use them if they are available in your workplace. ●

chair lift a technique for moving an ill or injured person down stairs or out of a building.

Figure 5.5 The stair chair is a commercial device designed to move ill or injured persons down stairs.

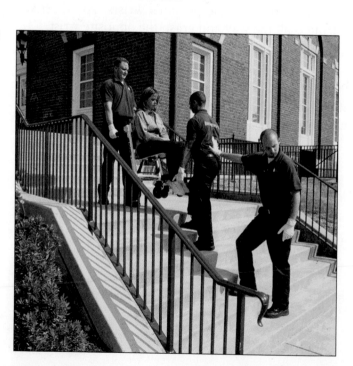

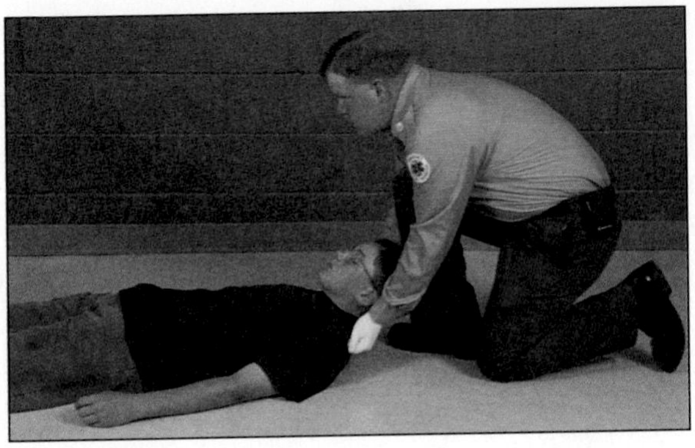

Figure 5.6 Clothes drag.

3. The second responder should kneel down in front of the person, facing her and grabbing onto the front legs of the chair.

4. Together both responders must lean the chair back and raise the chair off the ground.

5. Once both responders are standing comfortably, holding the chair with the person's feet forward, they can proceed toward the exit.

6. Use a third person as a spotter. Have him walk ahead of the responder at the feet of the person.

Clothes Drag

The **clothes drag** is an emergent move that is ideal for a single responder who must try to move an ill or injured person who is on the ground in an emergent situation. This is most often used as an emergent move since you would normally wait for additional help to move the person. Follow these steps to perform a clothes drag (▲ Figure 5.6):

clothes drag an emergent move; a technique by which a single responder can move an ill or injured person who is on the ground.

1. Kneel down at the head of the person.

2. Grab onto the clothing at the shoulders on each side.

3. Slowly raise up the person using his clothing. Pull him over the floor, making sure to drag along the long axis of the body.

THE HANDOFF

Fearing that the entire vehicle soon could be engulfed in flames, you quickly kneel at the man's head, grab his shirt tightly at the shoulders, and drag him backward away from the car. Once at a safe distance, you lay him back onto the pavement and quickly don exam gloves so you can apply pressure to a large laceration over his left ear and manually stabilize his head.

"What happened?" The man looks up at you, confusion softening his expression.

"You were in a car crash, sir." You hear sirens approaching. "Just don't move. Help is on the way."

The scene soon is awash in flashing red and blue lights, and you are relieved by the sounds of doors slamming, radios buzzing, and boots approaching you. Within moments, a firefighter assumes stabilization of the person's head and you step away as a coordinated group in uniforms swarms around the injured man. You see other firefighters rushing to extinguish the car, which is now fully engulfed in bright, rolling flames.

"You did a great job," an EMT says to you as he adjusts the straps on the backboard. "Thank you."

As you walk back toward the mall entrance, you are filled with pride at having the opportunity to make a difference in somebody's life.

CHAPTER REVIEW

Chapter Summary

- Learning and using proper body mechanics is important to minimize injury to both responders and the person being moved.

- In most instances you will want to leave an ill or injured person as you find him, but there may be times when it is necessary to move him before EMS arrives. You may decide to move a person if he is in imminent danger of further harm or if you are unable to provide the care he needs in the position in which you find him.

- You must learn and use proper body mechanics to minimize injury to yourself, anyone assisting you, and the ill or injured person.

- Characteristics of proper body mechanics include utilizing the right amount of people for the lift, keeping your feet shoulder width apart, lifting with your legs and not with your back, keeping your back as straight as possible, and keeping the weight of the person as close to you as possible.

- The risks of not using proper body mechanics can range from simple muscle pulls to severe injury to one's back. It can also result in further injury to the person in your care.

- One of the most important safety tips for a successful lift is good verbal and visual communication before, during, and after each move or lift.

- Emergent moves should be used whenever the ill or injured person is at risk of further injury and it is safe for the responder to move her quickly. Another reason for an emergent move is any immediate problem with the airway, breathing, circulation, or bleeding.

- The recovery position is used to assist in maintaining an open and clear airway. It is used only when you do not suspect a neck or back injury.

- Some of the most common techniques used to move ill or injured people are the log roll, extremity lift, chair lift, and clothes drag.

Quick Quiz

1. You are the only Emergency Responder at the scene of a man who has rolled over in a forklift. He was thrown from the forklift and is lying unresponsive on the ground. There is a full, unsecured pallet on the shelf overhead that looks like it might fall at any moment. If you felt it was safe to approach the person, what should you do next?

   a. Perform an extremity lift.

   b. Perform a clothes drag.

   c. Wait for additional help to arrive.

   d. Perform a chair lift.

2. Proper body mechanics include keeping your feet shoulder width apart, keeping the weight as close as possible, and:

   a. lifting with your legs.

   b. keeping your back bent.

   c. leaning as far over the person as possible.

   d. twisting at the hips and not the shoulders.

3. The risks of NOT using proper body mechanics when moving and lifting are possible injury to yourself and:

   a. damage to the chair.

   b. inability to maintain a proper airway for the person.

   c. an increased chance of dropping the person.

   d. a decreased chance of dropping the person.

4. The recovery position is MOST appropriate for which one of the following people?

   a. Responsive person who is not breathing adequately

   b. Unresponsive fall victim with a possible neck injury

   c. Unresponsive person who has no pulse

   d. Unresponsive person who is breathing adequately

5. Which one of the following moves would be most appropriate for an elderly ill or injured person who is having difficulty breathing and must be evacuated from the second floor of a building?

   a. Log roll

   b. Extremity lift

   c. Chair lift

   d. Clothes drag

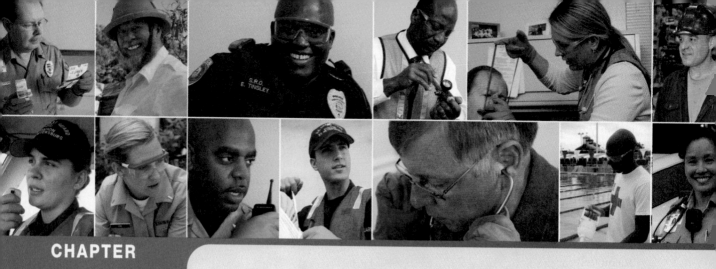

CHAPTER

6

Airway Management and Rescue Breathing

KEY TERMS

The following terms are introduced in this chapter:

- respiration *(p. 68)*
- respiratory arrest *(p. 69)*
- respiratory difficulty *(p. 68)*
- ventilations *(p. 70)*

LEARNING OBJECTIVES

At the conclusion of this chapter and the associated instructor-guided lesson, the student will be able to:

Cognitive

6.1 Describe the signs of an open and clear airway. *(p. 62)*

6.2 Describe the signs of a complete and partial airway obstruction. *(p. 63)*

6.3 Explain the steps for managing a responsive person with a complete or partial airway obstruction. *(p. 63)*

6.4 Describe the signs and symptoms of normal and abnormal respirations. *(p. 68)*

6.5 Explain the common causes of respiratory difficulty. *(p. 68)*

6.6 Describe the signs and symptoms of respiratory difficulty. *(p. 69)*

6.7 Differentiate between respiratory difficulty and respiratory arrest. *(p. 69)*

6.8 Describe the steps for caring for a person with respiratory difficulty. *(p. 70)*

6.9 Explain the indications for rescue breathing. *(p. 70)*

6.10 Describe the various methods and tools available for providing rescue breathing. *(p. 70)*

6.11 Describe the signs of adequate rescue breathing. *(p. 71)*

Psychomotor

6.12 Demonstrate the proper use of the head-tilt/chin-lift maneuver.

6.13 Demonstrate the proper use of the jaw-thrust maneuver.

6.14 Demonstrate the proper technique for providing rescue breaths for an ill or injured person with abnormal respirations.

6.15 Demonstrate the proper management of a responsive person with a complete or partial airway obstruction.

Introduction

As you know, not all illnesses and injuries are life threatening. One of the most important skills you can develop as an Emergency Responder is how to prioritize illnesses and injuries and provide care accordingly. An area that is always a high priority is that of airway and breathing. The loss of an open airway or the inability to breathe normally can quickly lead to death. This chapter discusses the common causes of airway blockage and difficulty breathing and what you can do to manage both.

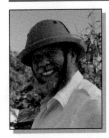

THE EMERGENCY

You step out of your truck and stand in the cool morning air, inhaling the fresh evergreen scent of the trees around you. As you look out across the misty lake, smooth and flawless like glass, reflecting the pink sky above, you are so grateful that you are working as a state park ranger this summer. A large fish splashes in the lake several feet from the shore and, as you are watching the widening ripples in the water, you hear a scream from the camping area nearby.

"Help!" A teenage girl is running barefoot across the parking lot toward you. "My dad is turning blue! Please help!"

You call for a medical response on the truck radio, grab the medical bag, and follow the girl as she turns and sprints back across the pavement and into the trees on the far side of the lot.

"What happened?" you ask, catching up to the girl near a green and white nylon tent.

"He's diabetic and I couldn't wake him and I was shaking him and he just started turning blue." Tears are running down her cheeks as she pulls the tent flap open.

You look into the dim interior of the tent and see a large, bearded man lying supine, eyes partially open, and the skin of his face an unnatural blue-gray.

AIRWAY MANAGEMENT

The body needs a constant supply of oxygen to survive. The air we breathe is made up of approximately 21 percent oxygen and 79 percent nitrogen, and this is more than enough to meet the daily demands for the majority of us. There are three conditions that are essential to ensure that we get the necessary supply of oxygen that our bodies need: an open and clear airway, an adequate volume of air with each breath, and a normal breathing rate (breaths per minute). Should an ill or injured person experience difficulty with any of these three factors, breathing will become compromised. The good news is that with proper training, Emergency Responders can help with each of these problems.

An Open and Clear Airway

6.1 Describe the signs of an open and clear airway.

The airway is made up of the areas at the back of the mouth and nose and includes the trachea (windpipe) (▼ Figure 6.1). When these areas are free of all obstructions, the airway is said to be open or clear. A person who is breathing effortlessly, silently, and with even rise and fall of the chest has an open and clear airway.

Many things can enter the airway, causing an obstruction and thus reducing the flow of air in and out. Common airway obstructions include the tongue, food, blood, saliva, and any small object that might have been swallowed. Obstructions can be either complete or partial. A complete obstruction prevents any air from moving through the airway and must be corrected immediately. Partial obstructions still allow for some movement of air through the airway and are typically not as life threatening. However, a partial obstruction can quickly become a complete one, so pay close attention to the person's ability to move air. If a partial obstruction does become complete, act quickly to remove it.

QUICK CHECK

Which problem requires the most immediate response— a partial airway obstruction or a complete obstruction? Explain your reasoning. ●

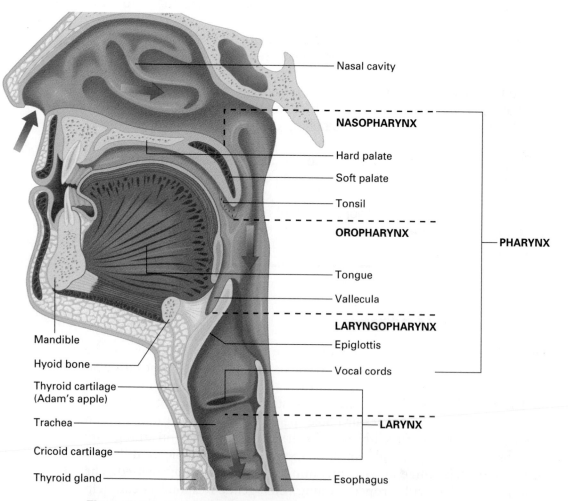

Figure 6.1 Anatomy of the upper airway.

Complete Airway Obstruction

Signs of a complete airway obstruction in a responsive person include the inability to breathe, cough, or speak. The person will appear panicked and may be grasping or pointing to his own throat in an attempt to alert you to what is happening. This is a true emergency and must be cared for immediately.

 PEDIATRIC CARE

One of the biggest differences between adults and children is the size of the airway. Due to the small size of a child's airway, it is much more prone to obstruction. ●

The care for a complete airway obstruction for a responsive person involves providing quick upward thrusts over the upper abdomen. These are referred to as abdominal thrusts.

Follow these steps to provide abdominal thrusts to a person with a complete obstruction (▼ Figure 6.2):

1. Ask the person if he is choking. If he cannot breathe, cough, or speak, you have confirmed a complete obstruction.

6.2 Describe the signs of a complete and partial airway obstruction.

6.3 Explain the steps for managing a responsive person with a complete or a partial airway obstruction.

Figure 6.2 Proper positioning for abdominal thrusts.

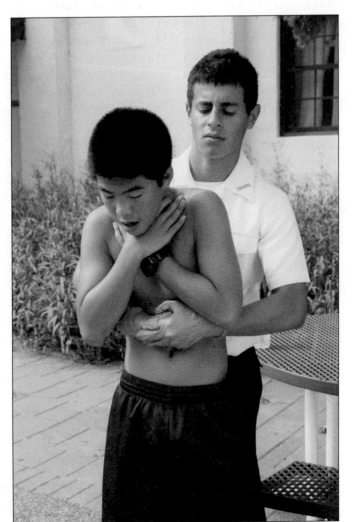

2. Stand directly behind the person and place one hand in the form of a fist right above his belly button. Your fist should be placed tightly against the abdomen with the thumb side in.

3. Next, reach around with the other hand and grasp your fist, pulling it tightly against the person's abdomen. Be sure your elbows are out and not pulled tightly against the person's sides.

4. Then, pull inward and upward sharply in separate and distinct thrusts. Be certain that you are not hitting any ribs as you thrust. Continue these thrusts one after the other until you relieve the obstruction.

Anyone who has received abdominal thrusts should be evaluated by a physician. Abdominal thrusts have been associated with serious injury to internal organs.

Partial Airway Obstruction

The signs of a partial airway obstruction are a little different from a complete obstruction. In many cases the person can still speak, but it may be difficult. He may only be able to speak in short one- or two-word sentences, and he may be somewhat panicked as well and will likely be coughing in an effort to remove the object from the airway.

The care for a person with a partial airway obstruction starts out a little less aggressively than care for a complete obstruction. In most cases, the person will be coughing. This is nature's way of clearing the obstruction, and it works quite well. Your job will be to recognize that there is a problem, confirm that it is only a partial obstruction, and encourage the person to cough forcefully. Confirming it as a partial obstruction is as simple as verifying that the person can produce a cough or speak at all.

Your job at this point is to encourage the person to produce strong, forceful coughs. You will want to remain close to him and evaluate his ability to produce a forceful cough. If he is unable to speak or unable to produce good forceful coughs, you may have to begin care as if the blockage were a complete obstruction, as described earlier. In this case, the person is clearly unable to move an adequate amount of air and eventually will become unresponsive. Your goal is to help him clear the obstruction before it gets to this point.

Once the obstruction has been cleared, it is important to remain with the person and observe him for an hour or so. Remember, anyone who has received abdominal thrusts should be evaluated by a physician.

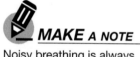

MAKE *A NOTE*

Noisy breathing is always a sign of a partial airway obstruction. ●

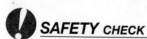

SAFETY CHECK

Managing a person's airway has its risks. As an Emergency Responder, you may be exposed to fluids such as saliva, blood, and vomit. So it is especially important that you wear appropriate protective equipment, such as gloves, a mask, and eye protection. ●

Managing the Airway of the Unresponsive Person

What if the person you are caring for is unresponsive? Is it possible to manage his airway properly and ensure that he is breathing normally? Certainly.

One thing is for certain: It is nearly impossible to provide rescue breaths to a person who is not lying face up. With that said, if you are not sure that the person you are caring for is breathing, roll him onto his back to assess airway and breathing status.

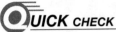

QUICK CHECK

For you to perform an adequate airway and breathing check of an ill or injured person who is unresponsive, what position must the ill or injured person be in? ●

First, confirm unresponsiveness by tapping the patient and shouting, "Are you okay"? Observe the patient for signs of absent or gasping breathing. If there is no chest movement or the patient is displaying only gasping breaths, consider his breathing inadequate (▼ Figure 6.3).

Head-Tilt/Chin-Lift Maneuver

Follow these steps to perform a head-tilt/chin-lift maneuver (▼ Figure 6.4):

1. Kneel down beside the person's head.
2. Place the palm of one hand on the person's forehead and two fingers of the other hand under the bony part of her chin.
3. With equal pressure on both hands, gently lift her chin and tilt her head backward.

Since the tongue is attached to the lower jaw, tilting the head back and lifting the chin will lift the tongue off the back of the throat and open the airway.

Jaw-Thrust Maneuver

In situations where you suspect that the person might have a neck or back injury, the jaw-thrust maneuver should be your first choice for attempting

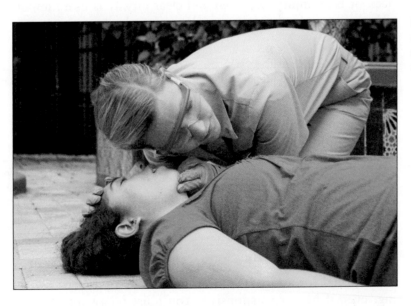

Figure 6.3 Maintaining an open airway in an unresponsive person who is breathing normally.

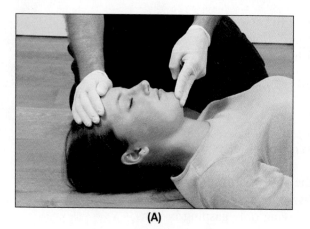 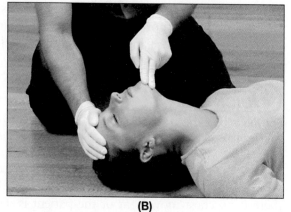

(A)   (B)

Figure 6.4 Use the head-tilt/chin-lift maneuver to open the airway if no neck or back trauma is suspected. (A) First, position your hands. (B) Then tilt the person's head back as far as it will comfortably go.

to open the airway. Follow these steps to perform a jaw-thrust maneuver (▶ Figure 6.5):

1. Kneel down at the top of the person's head.
2. Place your thumbs on her cheek bones while grasping the corners of her jaw with the first three fingers of each hand.
3. With gentle pressure, pull upward at the corners of her jaw, causing it to move forward.

By bringing the jaw forward you will lift the tongue off the back of the throat, thus clearing the airway. This is a difficult maneuver to perform, especially if it is necessary to provide rescue breaths for the person. If you are unable to adequately maintain an open airway using the jaw-thrust maneuver, you must move to the head-tilt/chin-lift maneuver, regardless of neck or back injury. An open and clear airway is more important than the risk of causing further injury to the neck or back.

QUICK CHECK

Should a head-tilt/chin-lift ever be attempted on a person with a suspected neck or back injury? Explain your answer. ●

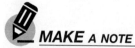

MAKE A NOTE

If you are unable to maintain an adequate airway using the jaw-thrust maneuver, you MUST use the head-tilt/chin-lift maneuver to ensure an open and clear airway. Ensuring an open airway and normal breathing is more important than the risk of making a neck or back injury worse. ●

Clearing the Airway

It is normal for an ill or injured person to experience nausea and vomiting, even if he is unresponsive. You must be aware of and prepared for

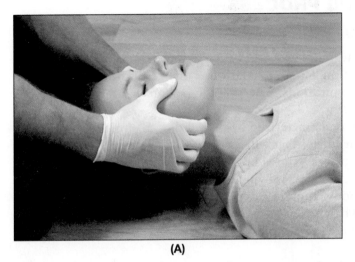

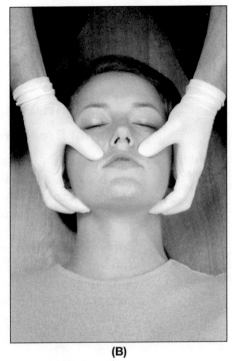

| (A) | (B) |

Figure 6.5 Use the jaw-thrust maneuver if you suspect neck or back trauma. (A) Side view. (B) Front view.

this possibility. Providing rescue breaths may even increase the chances that the person will vomit. This is not a bad sign, but it is one that must be managed quickly. If a person you are caring for begins to vomit, you must quickly roll him onto his side to allow for the vomit to exit the mouth and minimize the chances for it to enter the airway (▼ Figure 6.6).

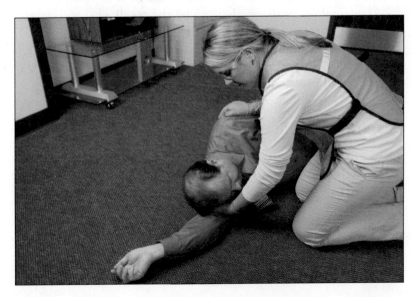

Figure 6.6 If a person you are caring for begins to vomit, you must quickly roll him onto his side.

In the best of circumstances, you will have plenty of help to roll the person should he vomit, but it may be necessary for you to roll a person onto his side by yourself.

THE BREATHING PROCESS

Normal Breathing

respiration one inhalation plus one exhalation of breath; also the exchange of oxygen and carbon dioxide at the cellular level.

Breathing is a very natural process that occurs approximately 18,000 times each day. One inhalation + one exhalation = one **respiration**. Breaths are often referred to as respirations. The average person breathes between 12 and 20 times per minute.

Normal breathing is characterized by the gentle and effortless movement of air in and out of the lungs. You will see only slight movement of the chest and/or abdomen of a person who is breathing normally. When everything is working normally and the air is moving in and out of the lungs properly, the oxygen enters the bloodstream deep within the lungs and carbon dioxide is removed with each exhalation. This exchange of oxygen and carbon dioxide is essential to life and is referred to as respiration.

6.4 Describe the signs and symptoms of normal and abnormal respirations.

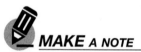

MAKE A NOTE

A person who is breathing normally often shows very little movement of the chest or abdomen. To the untrained eye, this could appear abnormally shallow, when in actuality it is quite normal. You can practice assessing normal breathing by quietly observing the breathing pattern of someone watching television, reading, or sleeping. ●

Abnormal Breathing

Abnormal breathing may be characterized as breathing that is too fast or too slow. Someone who is conscious and alert but experiencing difficulty breathing will have an increased work of breathing and an increased breathing rate. "Work of breathing" is the amount of effort necessary to breathe. Normal respirations are easy and effortless. Breathing that takes effort and is difficult is often referred to as **respiratory difficulty**, or shortness of breath. Signs of increased work of breathing include the use of abdominal and neck muscles to help move air in and out. If the person does not receive proper care promptly, he could experience respiratory arrest. Respiratory arrest can lead to, or be a sign of, cardiac arrest.

respiratory difficulty an increased work of breathing and an increased breathing rate; also called shortness of breath.

Abnormal respirations also can be the result of someone not breathing at an appropriate rate and/or volume. This can be caused by many things such as the fatigue of being in respiratory distress for too long, or the result of a drug overdose. It is important for you to be able to recognize both situations and provide the appropriate care until EMS arrives.

Respiratory Difficulty

6.5 Explain the common causes of respiratory difficulty.

Even with a clear and open airway, a person can experience respiratory difficulty. This can be the result of a variety of causes. Common causes of respiratory difficulty (shortness of breath) include the following:

- Asthma
- Heart attack
- Chemical exposure

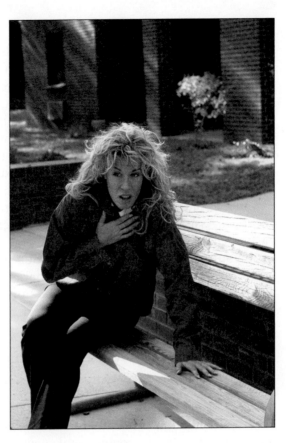

Figure 6.7 Shortness of breath is a sign of respiratory difficulty.

QUICK **CHECK**

What are the signs and symptoms of respiratory difficulty? ●

- Lung disease
- Allergic reaction

In most instances it will be easy to spot a person with respiratory difficulty (▲ Figure 6.7). Such a person often looks like someone who just ran the 100-yard dash and is trying catch his breath following the run. The biggest difference is that he typically has not been exerting himself and he does not get better by stopping the activity or resting. In many cases, the respiratory difficulty will continue to worsen unless he gets more advanced care.

6.6 Describe the signs and symptoms of respiratory difficulty.

Signs and symptoms of respiratory difficulty include the following:

- Increased breathing rate
- Increased work of breathing
- Panicked look
- Obvious movement of chest and abdomen
- Use of neck muscles to breathe

6.7 Differentiate between respiratory difficulty and respiratory arrest.

If someone with respiratory difficulty does not receive the appropriate care in a timely manner, it is possible that he would eventually go into respiratory arrest. **Respiratory arrest** is the complete stoppage of any attempts to breathe. Respiratory arrest can lead to, or be a sign of, cardiac arrest. This is a true emergency and must be cared for immediately if the person is to have any chance of survival.

respiratory arrest the complete stoppage of any attempts to breathe.

Caring for Respiratory Difficulty

6.8 Describe the steps for caring for a person with respiratory difficulty.

Managing a person with respiratory difficulty can be very stressful for both the person and the responder. Some of the basics are offered below. More detail is provided in Chapter 8, Caring for Medical Emergencies.

First and foremost, you must remain calm and do what you can to help calm the person who is having respiratory difficulty. Reassure him by telling him that additional help is on the way. Allow him to assume a position that is most comfortable for the situation. Do not try to make him lie down if he does not want to. In most cases he will already be in the position that is most comfortable for his situation. Ask if there is anything you can do to make him more comfortable. Loosen any restrictive clothing, such as collars or neckties. Assist him with taking any prescribed medication that he may have, such as an inhaler.

If you are trained in the administration of oxygen, then follow your local protocols and provide oxygen as appropriate. The administration of oxygen will be discussed in detail in Appendix 2 of this textbook.

Follow these guidelines when caring for a person with respiratory difficulty:

1. Activate 911.
2. Remain calm and provide lots of reassurance.
3. Assist the person with getting into a position of comfort.
4. Loosen any restrictive clothing.
5. Assist with medication as appropriate.
6. If trained to do so, provide supplemental oxygen. (Follow local protocols.)

ABSENT OR ABNORMAL BREATHING

6.9 Explain the indications for rescue breathing.

If you determine that an unresponsive person is not breathing or is only occasionally gasping, check for a pulse in the neck. If you definitely do not feel a pulse within 10 seconds, begin CPR with chest compressions. If an obvious pulse is present, provide rescue breaths. Occasional gasps are not normal and are not capable of supplying the person with enough oxygen to sustain life. Rescue breaths are artificial breaths that you give to a person by placing your mouth over an appropriate mask or barrier and blowing into the person's lungs. Rescue breaths help keep a person oxygenated. Rescue breaths are also called **ventilations**.

ventilations rescue breaths.

 MAKE A NOTE

You are probably wondering, "How is it possible to keep someone alive with my exhaled breaths?" You may remember that room air has approximately 21 percent oxygen concentration. Even after you have inhaled, your exhaled breath still has approximately 16 percent oxygen concentration. This is definitely enough to keep someone alive until he can receive more advanced care. ●

6.10 Describe the various methods and tools available for providing rescue breathing.

There are at least three methods available for providing rescue breaths. You must choose a method for which you were trained and the one that provides the best ventilations for the ill or injured person.

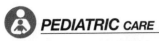

PEDIATRIC *CARE*

Children will breathe faster and move less volume than an adult will. Therefore, if you must provide rescue breaths, breathe more frequently (once every three to five seconds) and provide less volume (just enough to see the chest rise with each breath). ●

Rescue breaths should be provided at a rate of one breath every five to six seconds for an adult and every three to five seconds for a child.

When providing rescue breaths, it is common for some of the air being blown in to enter the stomach instead of the lungs. This can cause the person to vomit, can limit lung movement, and can reduce the effectiveness of rescue breathing. Providing breaths slowly over one second helps to keep down the pressure inside the throat and will minimize the chance for air to enter the stomach. Give enough air to make the chest visibly rise, but no more than that.

6.11 Describe the signs of adequate rescue breathing.

Methods for Providing Rescue Breaths

There are three methods that an Emergency Responder can use to provide rescue breaths: mouth-to-barrier-device ventilation, mouth-to-mask ventilation, and bag-mask ventilation. The bag-mask ventilation technique is described in Appendix 2.

A barrier device is any device used to protect the Emergency Responder from making direct contact with the skin of the person who needs breathing assistance. Barriers are quite portable and come in many different shapes and sizes. A barrier device is typically a flat sheet of plastic or vinyl with a hole or valve at the center (▼ Figure 6.8). The responder simply places the barrier over the person's mouth and then places his own mouth directly over the barrier. Finally, while pinching the person's nose, the responder blows air through the barrier and into the person's mouth.

A mask typically covers the person's mouth and nose (▼ Figure 6.9). At the top of the mask is a one-way valve into which the responder blows air. The one-way valve prevents the person's exhaled air from being directed back toward the face of the responder. Because the mask is larger than a barrier, it takes two hands and a little more practice to use it effectively.

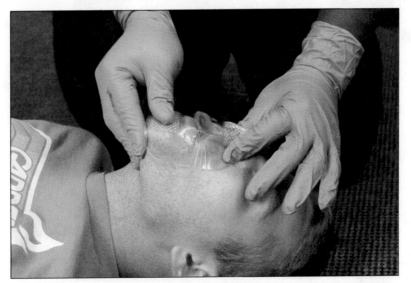

Figure 6.8 A barrier device is typically a flat sheet of plastic or vinyl with a hole or valve at the center.

Figure 6.9 Proper positioning for the facemask. (A) Place yourself beside the person's head. (B) Alternatively, position yourself directly above the head.

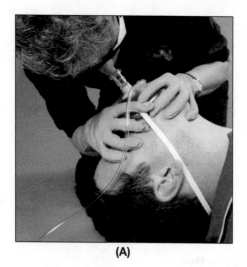

(A)

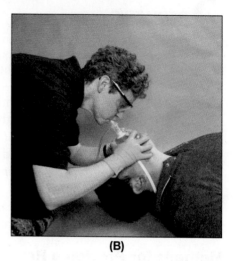

(B)

A bag mask is a much larger device and utilizes room air instead of the responder's own breath (▼ Figure 6.10). While it is possible for a single responder to use a bag mask, it is highly recommended that this device be used by two responders. With two responders, one uses both hands to ensure a good face seal with the mask, while the second responder squeezes the bag. The bag-mask technique is described in Appendix 2.

Figure 6.10 It is highly recommended that the bag-mask device be used with two responders. (A) Proper technique. (B) Proper hand placement.

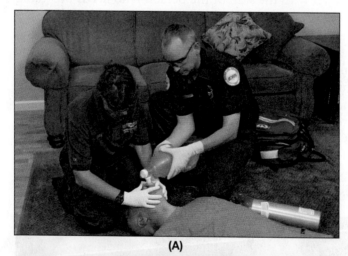

(A)

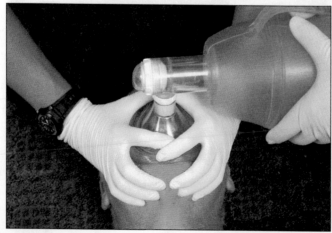

(B)

Providing Rescue Breaths

Follow these steps when providing rescue breaths for an unresponsive person who has a pulse but is not breathing or not breathing normally:

1. Position the person flat on his back.
2. Open the airway using the most appropriate method.
3. Confirm the patient is unresponsive, has a pulse, and is not breathing or has only gasping breaths.
4. Using an appropriate barrier device or mask, provide a rescue breath at the appropriate rate: one breath every five to six seconds for adults and every three to five seconds for a child. Each breath should last approximately one second.
5. Observe the chest for good rise and fall with each breath. Do not give too many breaths or breaths that are too large.
6. Reassess the pulse about every two minutes. If you do not feel a pulse within 10 seconds, begin CPR with chest compressions. Continue until EMS arrives and takes over.
7. If the person vomits, carefully roll him onto his side or turn his head to allow the vomit to exit the mouth. Use a gloved finger to sweep the mouth clear. Then roll the person onto his back and continue rescue breaths.

THE HANDOFF

You climb into the musty interior of the tent and kneel next to the man. The alarming blue-gray color of his face and lips is punctuated by abnormal noisy snoring with gasping breaths. You shake the man's shoulder, shouting for him to wake up. He responds with only a moan. You check his pulse and definitely feel it. You place your hand on his forehead and fingers under his jaw and tilt his head back, lifting his chin. He inhales suddenly and deeply. Almost immediately his skin color changes from blue-gray to pink.

"Oh, my gosh, thank you, thank you, thank you!" The girl yells from the tent entrance as you roll the still unresponsive man onto his side and wipe the sweat from your forehead. When the ambulance arrives at the campsite, the girl rushes off to meet the arriving crew.

You hear the girl outside the tent talking rapidly to the medics. "He's diabetic. He was blue and snoring and I couldn't wake him up. He gets like that sometimes when his sugar is low. The ranger saved him!"

"Okay, thanks. If that's the case then we'll just get him some glucose." You hear the voice of a paramedic named Ray who you just met last week during the park orientation. You then hear the rustle of fabric and feel a hand on your shoulder. Ray smiles at you when you look up.

"Great job, my friend!" he says, squatting next to the snoring man. "You remembered your basics, didn't you? And you just saved this man's life."

CHAPTER REVIEW

Chapter Summary

- An open and clear airway is essential to normal breathing. An open airway will allow for effortless breathing.

- An airway can be affected by either a complete or partial obstruction. A complete obstruction stops the flow of all air, while a partial obstruction allows for some air to move in and out of the lungs.

- It is important to act quickly and perform abdominal thrusts for a person experiencing a complete airway obstruction.

- People experiencing a partial airway obstruction should be encouraged to produce strong coughs in an attempt to remove the obstruction. If unsuccessful, it may be necessary to perform abdominal thrusts.

- Normal breathing is characterized by even and effortless breaths in and out at a normal rate. Abnormal breathing can be very fast and shallow, or very slow and gasping.

- Respiratory difficulty can be caused by many things. Some of the most common causes are asthma, heart attack, chemical exposure, lung disease, and allergic reaction.

- Signs and symptoms of respiratory difficulty include an increased breathing rate, increased work of breathing, panicked look, obvious movement of chest and abdomen, and the use of the neck muscles to breathe.

- Respiratory difficulty occurs when the body is trying to get more air and oxygen into the lungs. If this problem is not corrected, it can lead to respiratory arrest, which is the complete stoppage of all breathing effort. Respiratory arrest can lead to, or be a sign of, cardiac arrest.

- The following steps should be followed when caring for a person with respiratory difficulty:
  - Activate your emergency action plan or call 911.
  - Remain calm and provide lots of reassurance.
  - Assist the person with getting into a position of comfort.
  - Loosen any restrictive clothing.
  - Assist with medication as appropriate.
  - If trained, provide supplemental oxygen. (Follow local protocols.)

- The normal breathing rate for an adult is between 12 and 20 times per minute. If this rate becomes too slow, it may be necessary to provide rescue breaths (ventilations) for the person.

- Rescue breaths should be provided for anyone who is not breathing or who is not breathing normally. You can provide rescue breaths with a barrier device or mask. Breaths should be given at a rate of one breath every five to six seconds for an adult and every three to five seconds for a child.

- The best way to confirm that you are providing good rescue breaths is to observe for good rise and fall of the chest with each breath.

Quick Quiz

1. Signs of an open and clear airway include effortless breathing, silent breathing, and:

   a. good rise and fall of the chest.

   b. noisy breathing.

   c. use of the neck muscles.

   d. use of the abdominal muscles.

2. A person with a complete airway obstruction will NOT be able to:

   a. breathe, cough, or stand.

   b. breathe, cough, or speak.

   c. cough, speak, or stand.

   d. grab at his or her throat.

3. You are eating at a cafeteria and notice a woman across from you stand quickly and grab her throat. You approach her and ask if she can breathe or speak. She shakes her head no. What should you do next?

   a. Call 911.

   b. Provide rescue breaths.

   c. Provide abdominal thrusts.

   d. Ask her to cough forcefully.

4. Signs of abnormal breathing include all of the following EXCEPT:

   a. good rise and fall of the chest.

   b. gasping.

   c. chest rise.

   d. snoring.

5. You have been called to a man who was found slumped over in his office chair and unresponsive. You and another person carefully get the man to the floor. What should you do first?

   a. Give two slow rescue breaths.

   b. Perform a jaw-thrust maneuver.

   c. Look for normal breathing.

   d. Provide five abdominal thrusts.

6. All of the following are common causes of respiratory difficulty EXCEPT:

   a. suspected broken arm.

   b. asthma.

   c. heart attack.

   d. allergic reaction.

7. A person who presents with increased work of breathing can also be said to be experiencing:

   a. respiratory arrest.

   b. heart attack.

   c. brain attack.

   d. difficulty breathing.

8. A person who has stopped breathing on his own is said to be in:

   a. respiratory arrest.

   b. respiratory difficulty.

   c. shortness of breath.

   d. respiratory distress.

9. When providing rescue breaths for an adult, you should give:

   a. two breaths per minute.

   b. one breath every five to six seconds.

   c. one breath every three to five seconds.

   d. two breaths every five to six seconds.

10. You have assessed an unresponsive ill person and found her gasping. You definitely feel a pulse. What should you do next?

   a. Roll her onto her side.

   b. Provide abdominal thrusts.

   c. Encourage her to cough forcefully.

   d. Provide rescue breaths.

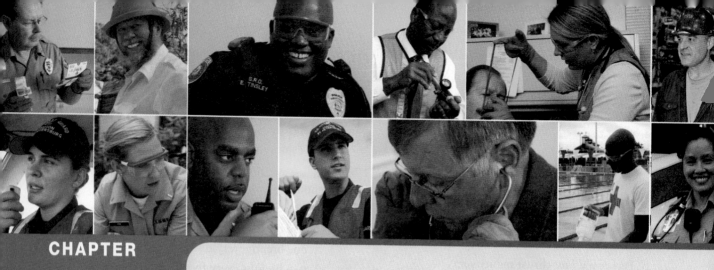

Principles of Assessment

KEY TERMS

The following terms are introduced in this chapter:

- chief complaint *(p. 84)*
- crepitus *(p. 85)*
- general impression *(p. 78)*
- immediate life threat *(p. 80)*
- mechanism of injury *(p. 78)*
- nature of illness *(p. 77)*
- primary assessment *(p. 80)*
- reassessment *(p. 92)*
- scene size-up *(p. 79)*
- secondary assessment *(p. 83)*
- sign *(p. 79)*
- symptom *(p. 79)*
- vital signs *(p. 87)*

LEARNING OBJECTIVES

At the conclusion of this chapter and the associated instructor-guided lesson, the student will be able to:

Cognitive

7.1 Differentiate between mechanism of injury and nature of illness. *(p. 77)*

7.2 Differentiate between a sign and a symptom. *(p. 79)*

7.3 Describe the components of an appropriate assessment and the purpose of each. *(p. 79)*

7.4 Describe the methods used to assess and quantify an ill or injured person's mental status. *(p. 81)*

7.5 Describe the components of the SAMPLE history tool. *(p. 83)*

7.6 Describe the components of the BP-DOC assessment tool. *(p. 84)*

7.7 State the characteristics that are obtained and measured when assessing respirations, pulse, and skin signs. *(p. 87)*

7.8 Describe the purpose and elements of the reassessment. *(p. 91)*

7.9 Explain the importance of documentation of all ill or injured person care. *(p. 92)*

Psychomotor

7.10 Demonstrate the ability to properly perform a scene size-up.

7.11 Demonstrate the ability to properly perform a primary assessment.

7.12 Demonstrate the ability to properly perform a secondary assessment.

7.13 Demonstrate the ability to properly obtain and document vital signs.

7.14 Demonstrate the ability to properly perform a reassessment.

7.15 Demonstrate the ability to properly identify and care for immediate life threats during an assessment.

Introduction

O*NE* of the most important skills you will learn and use as an Emergency Responder is the ability to properly assess an ill or injured person. A good assessment includes both the asking of questions related to the person's condition and the actual examination of the body when appropriate. It is safe to say that a good assessment will likely result in good care, while a poor assessment is more likely to result in poor care. Therefore, the skill of assessment is an important one. This chapter introduces the vocabulary associated with the assessment as well as the proper steps for completing a good assessment of an ill or injured person.

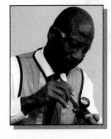

THE EMERGENCY

You are just finishing lunch when you hear a piercing tone over the factory loudspeakers followed by the operator's echoing voice. "Attention all Emergency Response Team members. Please respond to the level-two mezzanine." You have been on the company's Emergency Response Team for two months, and this is the first time that you have been summoned. Your heart begins racing and your hands shake slightly as you throw your sandwich wrapper and napkin into the garbage can on your way out of the lunchroom.

The level-two mezzanine, a plain concrete walkway overlooking the bustling production lines below, appears empty from your vantage point as the cargo elevator rumbles up to the main level. As the cage doors scrape open, you grab the red ERT bag from its place on the shelf and rush to the skeletal staircase leading to the mezzanine.

Reaching the top of the stairs, you see that Frank, the dayshift production supervisor, is lying on his back on the mezzanine.

"Thank heavens you're here!" Frank's assistant, Trina, runs up from the opposite end of the walkway. "We were talking and he just kind of slumped into the wall and passed out. I helped him to the floor and ran and called for help."

"Well, the scene is safe," you say to yourself, looking around the mezzanine and factory below. "It doesn't seem to be a trauma. Did he hit his head or twist his neck when you helped him to the ground?"

"No." Trina shakes her head vigorously. "I was really gentle."

You kneel next to Frank and immediately notice how pale his face is. "Frank!" you shout, gently shaking his shoulder. "Frank, I need you to wake up!"

There is no response, and as you lean down to check on Frank's breathing you instruct Trina to go get the defibrillator and make sure that the operator has contacted 911 to activate local EMS.

ILLNESS OR INJURY

All of the people whom you will be called upon to assist during an emergency may be categorized, at least initially, as either ill or injured. The **nature of illness** is the general nature of the person's chief complaint, such as difficulty

7.1 Differentiate between mechanism of injury and nature of illness.

nature of illness refers to the general nature of the ill person's complaint, such as difficulty breathing, chest pain, or dizziness.

Figure 7.1 The nature of illness refers to the general cause of the complaint, such as difficulty breathing, chest pain, or dizziness.

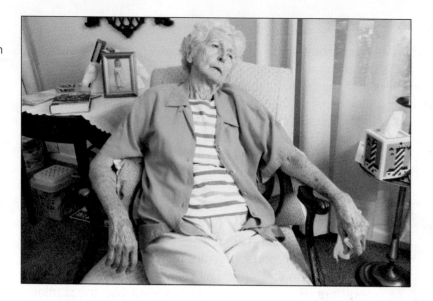

mechanism of injury refers to the general cause of a person's injury.

breathing, chest pain, or dizziness (▲ Figure 7.1). The **mechanism of injury** is the general cause of a person's injury (▼ Figure 7.2). For instance, a vehicle collision, a fall from a height, and a twisted ankle are all common mechanisms of injury.

Trained Emergency Responders generally evaluate how serious the situation is by how the person is acting or responding when they arrive on scene, but this is not always a reliable indicator for how serious things might be. You could have someone who is just lying there quietly and in very little distress but who is having a major heart attack and needing EMS assistance as soon as possible. On the other hand, you could arrive to find the person screaming in pain and only suffering from a twisted ankle, which is certainly not a life-threatening condition. So you see, when you first arrive on the scene of an emergency, you will need to use your best judgment and experience to form what is called a **general impression**.

general impression a quick assessment of the seriousness of the situation performed upon arrival at the scene.

A general impression is a quick assessment of the seriousness of the situation. You might ask yourself, "Is this a big problem requiring immediate 911

Figure 7.2 The mechanism of injury is the general cause of a person's injury.

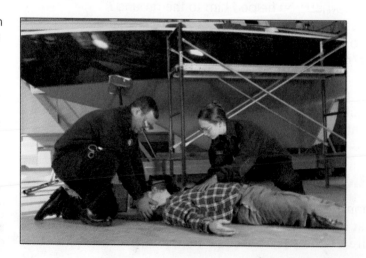

TABLE 7.1 Signs and Symptoms	
Signs	**Symptoms**
Something that you can see or measure, such as:	Something the person complains of or describes to you, such as:
• Bleeding • Swelling • Vital signs (heart rate, breathing rate, skin color)	• Pain • Nausea • Dizziness

assistance or something less serious so I can take a few minutes to assess the person and better determine what the needs might be?"

SIGNS AND SYMPTOMS

As you perform your assessment of the ill or injured person, you will be looking for anything that is wrong or anything that the person complains of or describes to you. These are called signs and symptoms (Table 7.1). A **sign** is something you can actually see or measure, such as bleeding, swelling, bruising, or how fast or slowly a person is breathing. You cannot see a **symptom**, but the ill or injured person feels it and can describe it to you, such as pain, nausea, or dizziness.

You will want to gather as much information about the problem or problems as possible, including performing a thorough visual and hands-on assessment of the person as well as asking very specific questions about the complaint. Together these tasks make up the assessment.

THE ASSESSMENT

A good assessment must be performed in a logical and consistent manner to help ensure that nothing is missed. For this reason, the assessment is broken down into the following components: scene size-up, primary assessment, and secondary assessment. The secondary assessment is made up of the history and physical examination, including vital signs, the reassessment, and documentation.

Scene Size-Up

The purpose of the **scene size-up** is to identify any immediate or potential hazards at the scene of the emergency as well as the need for additional resources. The scene size-up must be performed as you approach the scene and before you get too involved in caring for the ill or injured person (▼ Figure 7.3).

7.2 Differentiate between a sign and a symptom.

sign something that can be seen or measured, such as bleeding, swelling, bruising, or how fast or slow an ill or injured person is breathing.

symptom something that cannot be seen but the ill or injured person feels and can describe, such as pain, nausea, or dizziness.

QUICK CHECK

What is the term used to describe the general nature of a person's injury? Of a person's illness? ●

7.3 Describe the components of an appropriate assessment and the purpose of each.

scene size-up an overview of the scene of the emergency to identify any immediate or potential hazards at the scene as well as the need for additional resources.

Figure 7.3 The purpose of the scene size-up is to identify any immediate or potential hazards as well as the need for additional resources.

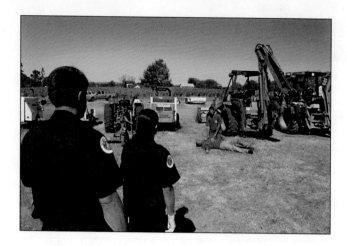

The scene size-up consists of the following components:

- **Safety.** This includes identifying any hazards at the scene, such as traffic, falling debris, toxic fumes, fire, threatening people, and so on. It also includes identifying the need for personal protection, such as gloves, mask, and eye protection.

- **Nature of illness or mechanism of injury.** You must do your best to determine if this is a medical complaint (illness) or a complaint related to an injury.

- **Number of ill or injured persons.** You must identify as best you can how many people might be involved. In most instances it will probably be only one person. If for any reason there are multiple victims, you will need to let the 911 dispatcher know so he or she can send the appropriate resources.

- **Additional resources.** You must determine the need for additional resources, such as the fire department, ambulance, and/or law enforcement. Then call for them. It is not always obvious if you will need additional resources, but the sooner you request them the sooner they can be there to help.

- **Possible neck or back injury.** Refer to the mechanism of injury and if there is any possibility that the person could have a neck or back injury. If so, you must keep the person still and manually stabilize the head and neck as best as you can. This will be discussed more later.

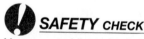 **SAFETY** CHECK

You are not obligated to help an ill or injured person if it puts you at risk. You must first do your best to ensure that all immediate risks have been mitigated before entering the scene. If you cannot mitigate a risk, do not enter the scene. Call 911 and wait for the appropriate resources to take over. ●

Primary Assessment

primary assessment the first step in the actual assessment of the ill or injured person; an examination that includes mental status, airway, breathing, circulation, and bleeding.

immediate life threat any condition that is immediately harmful to the ill or injured person, such as a blocked airway, inadequate breathing, or uncontrolled bleeding.

The objective of the **primary assessment** is to identify and care for any **immediate life threats** to the ill or injured person. Examples of immediate life threats include, but are not limited to, a blocked airway and anything that disrupts normal breathing or normal circulation, including severe bleeding. As long as it is safe to do so, you must address all immediate life threats when you find them.

The primary assessment is made up of the following components: mental status, airway status, breathing status, and circulatory status, including identifying severe, uncontrolled bleeding (Scan 7.1).

SCAN 7.1 Performing a Primary Assessment

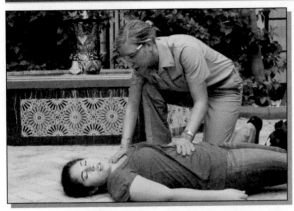

7.1.1 Tap and shout to assess for responsiveness. Look for normal breathing. If breathing is absent or not normal, such as only occasional gasps, assess circulation.

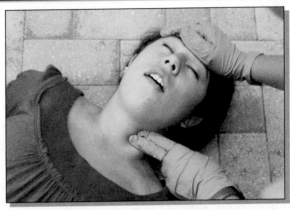

7.1.2 Check for a pulse. If you definitely do not feel a pulse within 10 seconds, begin CPR with chest compressions.

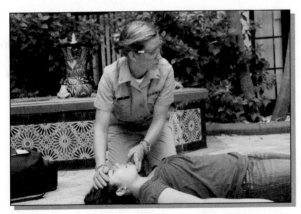

7.1.3 If an obvious pulse is present and the person is breathing normally, scan the body for major bleeding. If present, control the bleeding.

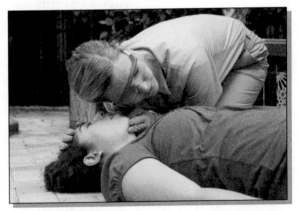

7.1.4 If the person has a pulse, is breathing normally, and there is no major bleeding, frequently reassess responsiveness, airway, breathing, and circulation until EMS arrives.

Mental Status

A person's mental status refers to his level of responsiveness and awareness of his surroundings and the situation. This is often one of the easiest things to determine as you approach the person. Begin by introducing yourself and see if the person responds in any way. You would expect a responsive person to look at you and respond verbally to your introduction.

7.4 Describe the methods used to assess and quantify an ill or injured person's mental status.

Is the person awake or unresponsive? If he is awake, then you will want to get a sense if he is alert or confused. This can provide insight into how bad things might be. A person who is alert and oriented to who he is, where he is, and the time of day is less urgent than someone who is confused. If the person is confused or disoriented in any way, this is evidence of a more serious underlying problem. Activate your emergency action plan or call 911.

An unresponsive person is one who appears to be unconscious and is not able to respond to your presence or your questions. You must rely on information from the scene and bystanders for clues as to what is going on with this person.

Below is a simple scale that can be used to help describe a person's mental status:

A – *Alert.* Address the patient, if he appears to be awake and spontaneously acknowledge you or answers back, he is *alert.*

V – *Verbal.* If the patient appears to be asleep or unconscious but responds to verbal commands or statements, this is considered *verbal.*

P – *Painful.* Pinch the patient's fingers or perform a sternal rub. If the patient awakens, responds verbally, or physically responds to this stimulus, this is *painful.*

U – *Unresponsive.* If the patient fails to respond verbally or physically to any of the above, he is *unresponsive.*

Airway Status

You have already learned that without an adequate supply of oxygen we would all die rather quickly. One part of ensuring that the ill or injured person can get an adequate supply of oxygen is to confirm that he has an open and clear airway. If the person is awake and talking, it is safe to assume that he has an open airway. However, if he is unresponsive, look for normal breathing.

Breathing Status

An open airway is only half the equation. To stay alive a person must be moving an adequate supply of air in and out of the lungs. In most cases, a person who is awake will be breathing adequately. It is the unresponsive person who needs a careful assessment of his breathing. Observe the person's breathing effort. Is it adequate or inadequate? Normal or abnormal? Look for normal rise and fall of the chest.

It may be difficult to determine if the person is breathing adequately. Occasional gasps are not normal and are not capable of supplying the person with enough oxygen to sustain life.

If for any reason you feel the person is not breathing adequately, you must provide rescue breaths.

Circulation Status

Circulation refers to two things. First is the flow of blood throughout the body. In other words, is the heart beating? You must check circulation by assessing for the presence of a carotid pulse in the neck. (See pages 87–88.)

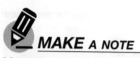

MAKE *A NOTE*

Mental status is not something you just assess once at the beginning of an assessment. It is a continuous process that occurs throughout your time with the person. Pay close attention to how the person responds to your questions and to the environment around him. Changes in responses may indicate that the person is getting worse or better. ●

The other is determining if there is any obvious uncontrolled bleeding that must be stopped. In most cases, if the unresponsive person is not breathing, or is only occasionally gasping and has no pulse, begin CPR, starting with chest compressions.

If the person is breathing normally, it is safe to assume that he has adequate circulation for the moment and you can move on to looking for and controlling any major bleeding. We will discuss more about how to control bleeding in Chapter 9.

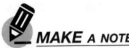

MAKE A NOTE

It is important to ensure that you have properly cared for any and all issues related to the primary assessment before you move on to the secondary assessment. You are not compelled to complete a secondary assessment if there are issues you must manage in the primary assessment. ●

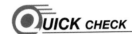

QUICK CHECK

Should you perform a primary assessment before or after the scene size-up? Explain your reasoning. ●

Secondary Assessment

The **secondary assessment** consists of two major components: the history, which is all the questions you want to ask about the problem, and the physical examination. In a perfect world, you will be able to perform both the history and the exam at the same time, but that really takes lots of practice. The secondary assessment is introduced here as a series of steps, so it will be easier to learn. With practice you will become more familiar with the flow of things, and the process will become more natural.

secondary assessment a thorough examination of the ill or injured person, beginning with the chief complaint and including evaluation of vital signs.

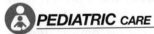

PEDIATRIC CARE

Beginning your assessment at the head can be very frightening for a child. In an effort to build trust, begin your assessment at the child's feet and work your way up to the head. Of course, if there are issues related to the ABCs (airway, breathing, circulation), you always would begin at the head. ●

History

You will want to find out as much as you can about what is going on with the ill or injured person during your assessment. This part of the assessment is called the history. The history includes as much information about the current problem or chief complaint and any past medical history that may pertain to the current situation. A helpful tool to help you remember the most important questions to ask is the SAMPLE acronym:

7.5 Describe the components of the SAMPLE history tool.

S – *Signs and symptoms.* Where does it hurt? How does it feel?

A – *Allergies.* Do you have any known allergies (food, bees, medications)?

M – *Medications.* Do you take any prescription or non-prescription medications? Have you taken them as prescribed?

P – *Pertinent medical history.* Do you have any existing medical history (diabetes, seizures, breathing problems, etc.)? Has this ever happened before?

L – *Last oral intake.* What is the last thing you had to eat or drink? When did you have it?

E – *Events leading to the call.* What were you doing when the incident (illness/injury) occurred? Did you do something that caused this to happen?

PEDIATRIC CARE

Children may not always be able to provide a detailed history of the situation or their condition. You may have to rely on family members or bystanders for much of the history. ●

QUICK CHECK

In what part of the SAMPLE history might you learn that the person you are caring for had a heart attack six months ago? ●

Physical Examination

There are generally two approaches to performing a physical assessment. The approach that you will take will be determined by the level of responsiveness of the ill or injured person.

SAFETY CHECK

Be sure to use protective gloves when performing a physical examination to protect against being exposed to blood or other body fluids. ●

Generally, a responsive person is able to talk to you and tell you what he is feeling, and he can answer your questions. Your assessment for a responsive person will be focused on the chief complaint. The **chief complaint** is the one thing that is causing the ill or injured person pain or discomfort. It is the reason for which help was called. You will focus your questions and physical exam on the chief complaint.

An unresponsive person cannot tell you what he or she is feeling. So you must rely on what you see during your physical examination and information you gather from bystanders.

MAKE A NOTE

Individual privacy must be considered at all times. Do your best not to expose an ill or injured person's body inappropriately. Sometimes it is best just to wait for EMS personnel to arrive. ●

chief complaint the one thing that is causing the ill or injured person pain or discomfort and is the reason for which help was called.

7.6 Describe the components of the BP-DOC assessment tool.

To perform a physical examination on an ill or injured person, use the BP-DOC assessment tool. It can help you remember what to look for:

B – *Bleeding.* You must observe and inspect for bleeding over the entire body, including areas that are difficult to see or reach, such as the back of the person.

P – *Pain.* Begin by asking the person if he has pain and where. You will then feel (palpate) for other areas that are painful as you perform your physical examination.

D – *Deformities*. Observe for deformities of any kind, such as angulated limbs, bumps, swelling, and so on.

O – *Open wounds*. Observe for any open wounds, especially wounds that may be bleeding.

C – *Crepitus*. **Crepitus** is a peculiar crackling or grating feeling or sound under the skin or in the joints. Recognizing this sound is especially important when you are examining an unresponsive person who cannot tell you he has pain. If you feel crepitus, you can assume there is an underlying bone or joint injury.

Using your gloved hands, carefully palpate (feel) each of the following areas of the body (Scan 7.2). It is important to be somewhat firm as you assess each area but not so firm that you cause the person unnecessary discomfort. Being too gentle will not reveal areas of pain and deformity that you

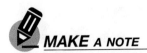

MAKE *A* **NOTE**

You will not perform a thorough physical examination of each area on every person. Your examination should be tailored to the needs of the ill or injured person based on several factors, such as mechanism of injury, nature of illness, chief complaint, and level of responsiveness. ●

crepitus a crackling or grating feeling or sound most commonly associated with broken bones.

SCAN 7.2   Secondary Assessment: The Physical Exam

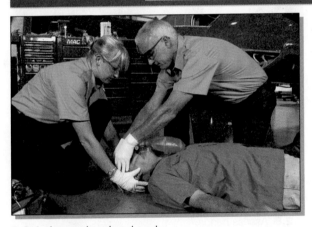

7.2.1 Assess head and neck.

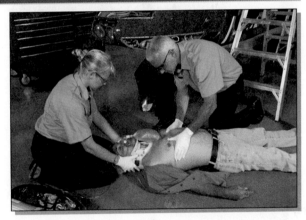

7.2.2 Assess chest.

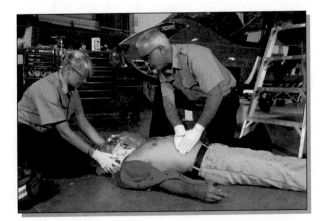

7.2.3 Assess abdomen.

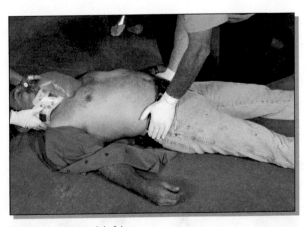

7.2.4 Assess pelvis/hips.

Continued on next page.

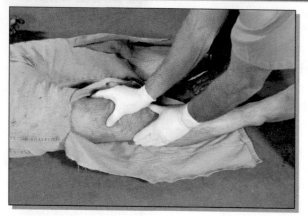

7.2.5 Assess legs.

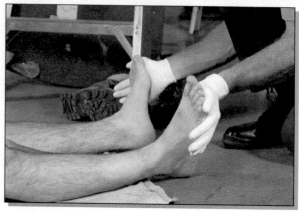

7.2.6 Assess feet.

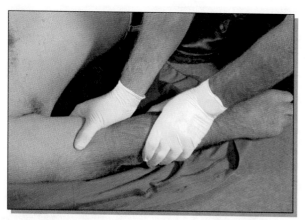

7.2.7 Assess arms.

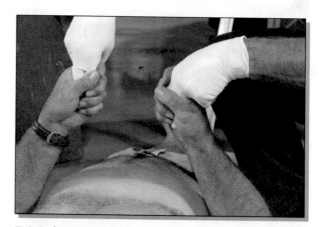

7.2.8 Assess hands.

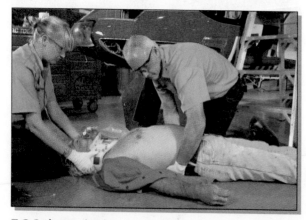

7.2.9 Assess back.

need to find. As you are doing so, also visually examine each area for anything abnormal.

- **Head/neck.** Assess for BP-DOC. If you find or suspect an injury to the head or neck, have another Emergency Responder (when available) use his or her hands to hold the person's head still. If you are alone, tell the person to keep his head and neck still before continuing to perform the physical examination.
- **Chest.** Assess for BP-DOC. Injuries to the chest can cause serious internal bleeding as well as breathing problems. Carefully monitor the breathing status of all those with chest injuries.
- **Abdomen.** Assess for BP-DOC. Pain in the abdomen could be a symptom of internal injury and/or bleeding.
- **Pelvis/hips.** Assess for BP-DOC. This is another area that can hide serious internal bleeding.
- **Legs/feet.** Assess for BP-DOC. If necessary, you may need to cut away clothing to get a better look at a painful area. This is especially important if blood-soaked clothing suggests serious, uncontrolled bleeding. If it is not painful to the person, remove the shoes and ask the person to move his feet. Ask if he can feel you touching his toes.
- **Arms/hands.** Assess for BP-DOC. If necessary, you may need to cut away clothing to get a better look at a painful area. Ask the person to move his hands and fingers.
- **Back.** Assess for BP-DOC. If possible, assess the back. You may not want to move the person to do this unless you have reason to believe there is serious, uncontrolled bleeding. If you must move the person, ask for assistance from others to keep the neck and back in alignment.

Vital Signs

An important component of any good assessment is the obtaining of the person's **vital signs**. Common vital signs that can be obtained and monitored without special equipment include the pulse, respirations, and skin signs.

Blood pressure also is considered a vital sign, but because taking a blood pressure requires the use of specialized equipment, it is covered in Appendix 1.

Pulse Points

A pulse is nothing more than a remote heartbeat. It is caused by the pressure inside the artery that occurs with each beat of the heart. It can be felt with the fingers when the pulse point lies close to the skin and over a hard structure such as a bone. The following are two of the most commonly used pulse points on the body:

- **Carotid pulse point.** This is found at the front of the neck immediately adjacent to the windpipe (trachea). This is the most common place to confirm the presence of circulation for an unresponsive person (Scan 7.3).

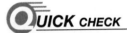

QUICK CHECK

Is the assessment process different or the same for an unresponsive person compared to a responsive person? Explain your reasoning. ●

7.7 State the characteristics that are obtained and measured when assessing respirations, pulse, and skin signs.

vital signs the key signs of life, which include respirations, pulse, skin signs, and blood pressure.

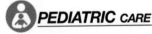

PEDIATRIC CARE

Vital signs can vary widely between adults and children. In general, breathing and pulse rates in children are faster and blood pressure is lower. ●

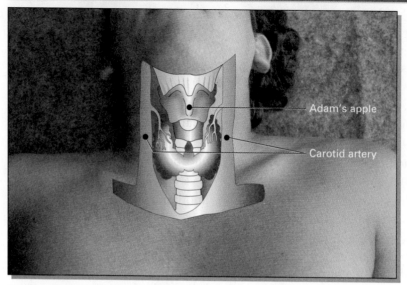

7.3.1 Locating the carotid artery.

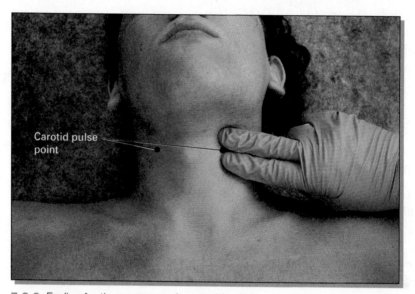

7.3.2 Feeling for the presence of a carotid pulse.

- **Radial pulse point.** This is found at the wrist of either arm. It is located on the anterior side of the wrist just proximal to the thumb. This is the most common pulse point used to confirm circulation when caring for a responsive person (Scan 7.4).

There are three characteristics you can measure when assessing a person's pulse: rate, strength, and rhythm. A normal pulse rate can range between 60 and 100 beats per minute. You will need a watch with a second hand or a digital watch to accurately record a person's pulse rate. Locate the

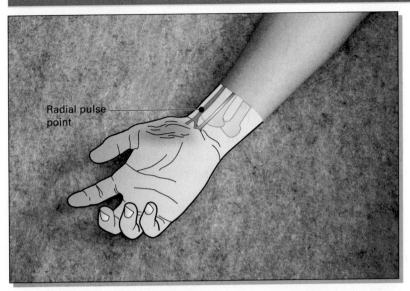

7.4.1 Locating the radial pulse point.

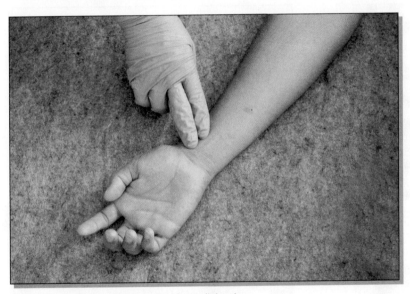

7.4.2 Feeling for the presence of a radial pulse.

appropriate pulse point and count the number of beats you feel for 15 seconds. Then multiply that number by four to get an accurate minute rate. Pulse rates are always described as a rate per minute.

At the same time you are counting the rate, you should be paying attention to how strong or weak the pulse feels and whether it is regular or irregular. These characteristics can be very subjective if you have only a little experience with taking pulses. Not to worry. If you can find a pulse and determine a minute rate, you are doing just fine.

Here are some different examples of how you might document a person's pulse: 72, strong and regular; 88, strong and irregular; 120, weak and regular.

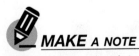

MAKE A NOTE

Do not use your thumb to locate the pulse of an ill or injured person. Your thumb has a pulse of its own and may be the pulse that you feel, rather than that of the person you are caring for. ●

Respirations

You may remember from the discussion in Chapter 6 that one inhalation plus one exhalation equals one respiration. Much like pulses, respirations have three characteristics that must be measured when evaluating respirations: rate, depth, and ease.

A normal respiratory rate is between 12 and 20 breaths per minute. The easiest way to measure respiratory rate is to watch the movement of the chest and abdomen with each breath. Remember, one inhalation plus one exhalation equals one respiration. Count the breaths for 15 seconds and multiply by four. This will give you the person's minute rate. It is advised that you not make it too obvious that you are counting respirations. Once a person becomes aware that you are counting respirations, he may inadvertently change his breathing rate (Scan 7.5).

As you are counting the rate, you also will want to observe the depth of each breath. It should be normal, which is sometimes described as shallow to the untrained eye. A person who is breathing with an adequate depth is said to be breathing with a good tidal volume (GTV).

| SCAN 7.5 | Assessing Respiration |

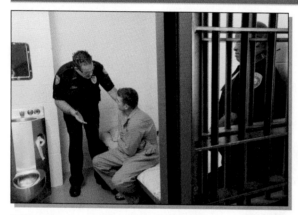

7.5.1 As you question the person about his chief complaint, notice if his breathing is labored or easy.

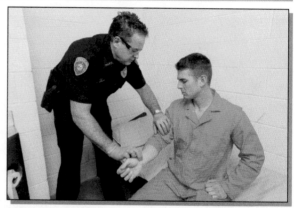

7.5.2 Locate the radial pulse, place the arm across the abdomen, and count the pulse for 15 seconds.

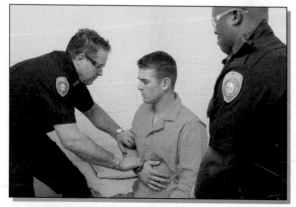

7.5.3 After you've taken the pulse, continue to hold the wrist as if you are still assessing the pulse.

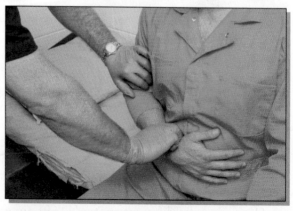

7.5.4 Then count respirations by seeing and feeling the rise and fall of the chest and abdomen.

You also will want to observe how easy or difficult it is for the person to take each breath. When it is difficult for a person to breathe, it is often referred to as labored respirations. Here are some examples of how you might document a person's respirations: 12, GTV, unlabored; 32, shallow, labored; 24, deep, labored.

Skin Signs

Skin signs are one of the easiest vital signs to observe when caring for an ill or injured person. They take no special equipment and often can be evaluated in a matter of seconds. You will assess the following skin signs: color, temperature, and moisture.

Normal skin signs of light-skinned individuals are described as pink, warm, and dry. When assessing the characteristics of dark-skinned individuals, look at the inside of the lower lip or the nail beds for color. These areas will appear pink in a person with normal skin signs.

Skin temperature can be affected by the environment or exertion, so you must take these factors into consideration. It is easiest to use the back of a bare hand or the wrist of your gloved hand to feel the forehead for temperature (Scan 7.6). It is quite simple to evaluate: It will be hot, warm, or cool to the touch.

Moisture also is affected by the environment and exertion, so keep that in mind. Normal skin is dry. Moist skin is typically not normal for a person at rest and may be a sign of stress on the body.

The following are some examples of how one might document a person's skin signs: pink, warm and moist; pale, cool, moist; flushed, hot, dry.

Reassessment

The assessment of an ill or injured person is never complete. Just when you come to the end of a secondary assessment it is time to go back to the beginning and perform another primary assessment. The process is a cycle that repeats itself as long as you are with the ill or injured person.

7.8 Describe the purpose and elements of the reassessment.

SCAN 7.6   Assessing Skin Signs

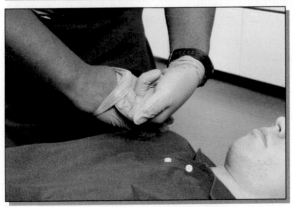

7.6.1 Pull down part of your protective glove to bare the back of your hand.

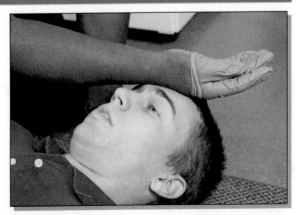

7.6.2 Place it on the ill or injured person's forehead to feel for temperature (hot, warm, or cool to the touch) and moisture.

reassessment a recheck of the ABCs, chief complaint, vital signs, and interventions.

A proper **reassessment** should be performed at regular intervals. It is recommended that you perform a reassessment every five to 15 minutes, depending on the condition of the person. The more serious the situation, the more frequent the reassessment should be. An ill or injured person's condition can change quickly. You want to be ready to adjust your care if the person's condition warrants it.

A proper reassessment should include the following elements:

- **Primary assessment.** Recheck the status of airway, breathing, and circulation (ABCs).
- **Chief complaint.** Reassess the chief complaint to determine if signs and symptoms appear to be getting better or worse or are remaining the same.
- **Vital signs.** A change in vital signs can be an indication that the person's condition is changing.
- **Interventions.** Interventions refer to the care that you are providing. Does your care seem to be helping the person feel better? If so, great. If not, then consider a change that might be better for the person. For example you may want to help the person into a position that is more comfortable.

In many instances you will be quickly handing off the person to EMS providers or someone else with a higher level of training. For this reason, you may not have enough time to perform a reassessment. Just keep in mind that continuous monitoring is necessary as long as you are with the ill or injured person.

Documentation

7.9 Explain the importance of documentation of all ill or injured person care.

Documentation is a part of your duties as an Emergency Responder. It may be done in many forms, including in writing and verbally. In many cases, your verbal report becomes the basis for how the next level of care manages the person. Whenever possible, you should document in writing important information that you gather during your assessment. Your written documentation should be as objective and factual as possible and should include information such as the person's name, age, chief complaint, signs, symptoms, vital signs, the care you provided, and the person's response to that care.

You may not be able to document all of this information in writing before the person leaves with the EMS team, but you should take the time to carefully document all the pertinent facts once the call is over and before you return to your normal duties. The documentation of care should include the following elements, at a minimum:

- Person's name
- Person's age
- Chief complaint
- Signs and symptoms
- Vital signs
- Pertinent medical history
- The care you provided
- The person's response to your care

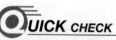

QUICK CHECK

Why is documentation important to the process of caring for a person who is ill or injured? ●

THE HANDOFF

You are on your third cycle of chest compressions on Frank when Trina scrambles back up to the mezzanine with the AED hanging over her shoulder, banging against her hip.

"The fire department is just coming up the elevator with the other ERT members," she says breathlessly. "They should all be here in a minute."

You continue chest compressions as Trina opens the AED, turns it on, and with shaking hands places the foam electrodes on the man.

"You're doing great," you say to her, taking deep breaths and sweating as the AED analyzes Frank's heart rhythm. "You put those pads on perfectly."

You hear a multitude of feet clumping up the stairs behind you as the AED voice says, "Shock advised." After it charges, you make sure that neither you nor Trina is touching Frank before pushing the large blinking button.

"What happened?" A firefighter squats next to you as the AED is analyzing Frank again.

"Uh, he was apparently just walking with Trina and passed out." You wipe sweat from your forehead with a gloved hand. "And when I got here he wasn't breathing and had no signs of life, so I started CPR and it shocked him once just now, and—"

"Resume CPR," the machine's automated voice interrupts you.

"We've got it." Two of the firefighters take over CPR as you stand to move out of their way.

Soon the AED demands a second shock. Afterward, incredibly, Frank moves his arm and begins to breathe on his own.

"That's amazing," Rhoann, a fellow member of your response team, whispers loudly into your ear as she grabs your arm. "You did such a great job. It looks like he is beginning to respond."

CHAPTER REVIEW

Chapter Summary

- All ill or injured persons can be categorized based on the mechanism of injury or nature of illness.

- Signs and symptoms are indicators that you will look for and evaluate as part of your assessment. A sign is something you can see, while a symptom is something the person tells you about the situation.

- The components of an assessment include the scene size-up, primary assessment, secondary assessment, and the reassessment. The scene size-up is mostly about safety and resources. The primary assessment is about identifying immediate life threats. The secondary assessment includes a physical examination and history. The reassessment includes reevaluating the assessment and any required interventions.

- Mental status can be assessed using the AVPU scale (alert, verbal, painful, unresponsive).

- The SAMPLE history tool stands for signs and symptoms, allergies, medications, past medical history, last oral intake, and events leading up to the incident.

- The BP-DOC assessment tool is used during the physical examination and stands for bleeding, pain, deformities, open wounds, and crepitus.

- Vital signs include respirations (rate, depth, ease), pulse (rate, strength, rhythm), and skin (color, temperature, moisture).
- The objective of the reassessment is to identify changes in the person's condition and evaluate the effectiveness of interventions.

- It is important to document all care provided to an ill or injured person. This helps to inform others who will be caring for the person and allows them to manage the person appropriately.

Quick Quiz

1. All of the following are examples of symptoms EXCEPT:
   a. nausea.
   b. cool skin.
   c. pain.
   d. fatigue.

2. Which one of the following describes the nature of illness?
   a. The person fell from a roof.
   b. The person has a badly twisted ankle.
   c. The person was struck in the head.
   d. The person is experiencing difficulty breathing.

3. Specific care that you provide to an ill or injured person is called a(n):
   a. intervention.
   b. assessment.
   c. initiative.
   d. scope.

4. Which one of the following is NOT usually considered part of the reassessment process?
   a. Asking permission to provide care
   b. Taking vital signs
   c. Evaluating the effectiveness of the treatment plan
   d. Checking the person's airway

5. Which one of the following lists the characteristics of a pulse?
   a. Speed, rate, threadiness
   b. Rate, strength, rhythm
   c. Regularity, tidal volume, rhythm
   d. Rate, depth, ease

6. The pulse point found on the anterior neck near the windpipe is called the _____ pulse point.
   a. distal
   b. pedal
   c. carotid
   d. radial

7. The O in the BP-DOC mnemonic stands for:
   a. open wounds.
   b. oral history.
   c. observable injuries.
   d. occlusions.

8. You are approached by a coworker who was injured during her lunch break. She tells you that her left wrist hurts and denies pain elsewhere. You should initially try to determine:
   a. the nature of her illness.
   b. what her medical history is.
   c. her chief complaint.
   d. the mechanism of injury.

9. You are at a family event and one of your relatives exclaims that he is too tired to continue playing catch with the football. As he walks over and slumps into a lawn chair, you notice that his breathing is rapid and his skin is pink and moist. Should you be concerned?
   a. Yes, these visual vital signs indicate that he is ill.
   b. No, because his appearance is consistent with his activity.
   c. Yes, because normal skin appearance should be pink and dry.
   d. No, because he does not have a chief complaint.

10. You arrive at the scene of a bicycle crash and find an unresponsive man lying on the pavement, blood oozing from his mouth and nose. What is the best way to determine if he has a pulse?
    a. Shake his shoulder and yell for him to respond.
    b. Feel for a radial pulse.
    c. The oozing blood indicates that he has circulation.
    d. Assess his carotid pulse point.

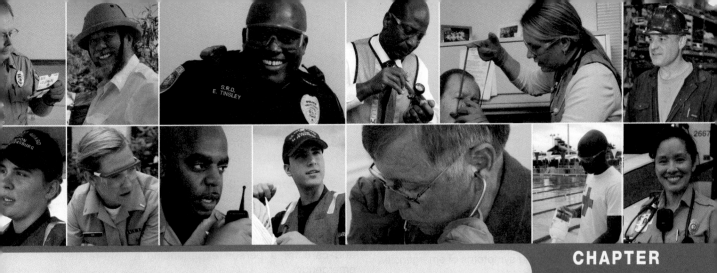

Caring for Medical Emergencies

LEARNING OBJECTIVES

At the conclusion of this chapter and the associated instructor-guided lesson, the student will be able to:

Cognitive

8.1 List the common signs and symptoms of a general illness. *(p. 97)*

8.2 Explain the steps for assessing an ill person. *(p. 98)*

8.3 Explain the common causes of altered mental status. *(p. 99)*

8.4 Describe the signs and symptoms of a person with an altered mental status. *(p. 100)*

8.5 Explain the appropriate care for a person with an altered mental status. *(p. 100)*

8.6 Describe the signs and symptoms of a person experiencing a generalized seizure. *(p. 100)*

8.7 Explain the appropriate care for a person experiencing a generalized seizure. *(p. 100)*

8.8 Describe the signs and symptoms of a person experiencing a stroke (brain attack). *(p. 101)*

8.9 Explain the appropriate care for a person experiencing a stroke (brain attack). *(p. 102)*

8.10 Describe the signs and symptoms of a person experiencing a diabetic emergency. *(p. 103)*

8.11 Explain the appropriate care for a person experiencing a diabetic emergency. *(p. 103)*

8.12 Describe the signs and symptoms of a person experiencing chest pain. *(p. 104)*

8.13 Explain the appropriate care for a person experiencing chest pain. *(p. 104)*

8.14 Describe the signs and symptoms of a person experiencing difficulty breathing. *(p. 105)*

8.15 Explain the appropriate care for a person experiencing difficulty breathing. *(p. 106)*

8.16 Describe the signs and symptoms of a cold-related emergency. *(p. 107)*

KEY TERMS

The following terms are introduced in this chapter:

- altered mental status *(p. 99)*
- angina *(p. 103)*
- brain attack (stroke) *(p. 101)*
- convulsions *(p. 100)*
- cyanosis *(p. 106)*
- diabetes *(p. 102)*
- epilepsy *(p. 100)*
- frostbite *(p. 107)*
- generalized seizure *(p. 100)*
- heart attack *(p. 103)*
- heat exhaustion *(p. 109)*
- heat stroke *(p. 108)*
- hypothermia *(p. 107)*
- overdose *(p. 110)*
- postictal *(p. 101)*
- tripod position *(p. 105)*

8.17 Explain the appropriate care for a person experiencing a cold-related emergency. *(p. 108)*

8.18 Describe the signs and symptoms of a person experiencing a heat-related emergency. *(p. 109)*

8.19 Explain the appropriate care for a person experiencing a heat-related emergency. *(p. 110)*

8.20 Describe the signs and symptoms of a person experiencing an overdose or poisoning. *(p. 110)*

8.21 Explain the appropriate care for a person experiencing an overdose or poisoning. *(p. 111)*

8.22 Describe the signs and symptoms of emergencies related to bites and stings. *(p. 111)*

8.23 Explain the appropriate care for a person experiencing an emergency related to a bite or sting. *(p. 112)*

Psychomotor

8.24 Demonstrate the ability to appropriately assess a person with a general medical complaint.

8.25 Demonstrate the ability to appropriately assess and care for a person with an altered mental status.

8.26 Demonstrate the ability to appropriately assess and care for a person experiencing a generalized seizure.

8.27 Demonstrate the ability to appropriately assess and care for a person experiencing a stroke (brain attack).

8.28 Demonstrate the ability to appropriately assess and care for a person experiencing a diabetic emergency.

8.29 Demonstrate the ability to appropriately assess and care for a person experiencing chest pain.

8.30 Demonstrate the ability to appropriately assess and care for a person experiencing difficulty breathing.

8.31 Demonstrate the ability to appropriately assess and care for a person experiencing a cold-related emergency.

8.32 Demonstrate the ability to appropriately assess and care for a person experiencing a heat-related emergency.

8.33 Demonstrate the ability to appropriately assess and care for a person experiencing an emergency related to a bite or sting.

8.34 Demonstrate the ability to appropriately assess and care for a person experiencing an overdose or poisoning.

Introduction

You have already learned that emergencies can be divided into two broad categories: illnesses and injuries. This chapter discusses some of the more common emergencies related to illness. Caring for a person with an illness can be a bit more challenging than caring for a person with an injury, especially when he is unresponsive and cannot tell you what might be wrong. As you will see, there are several common illnesses that can become emergencies if not managed properly. Some of them are discussed here, along with the signs and symptoms of each and the most appropriate care to provide.

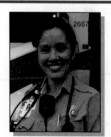

THE EMERGENCY

As you walk through the dim administrative segregation unit of the jail, you notice that the sunrise is just beginning to tint the frosted day room windows a pale yellow. You inhale deeply, knowing that walking down the line of heavy steel doors, knocking on them to wake the inmates for breakfast, is your last task before the end of your graveyard shift and the beginning of four days off.

"Let's go, gentlemen," you shout from door to door. "Chow time!"

As you pass door number 11 and peer into the small window, you notice that the inmate is staring out at you with a confused look in his eyes. You also see that the right side of his face is noticeably relaxed, drooping lower than the other side.

"Hey, Matt." You call your unit partner on the portable radio. "Can you pop 11 and call for the nurse?"

After hearing the thud of the magnetic lock releasing, you pull the door open and lead the limping inmate over to one of the stainless steel tables in the day room.

"Is everything okay, Hector?" you say while donning exam gloves.

"I was just swimming in my bed," he says earnestly and then points to his head. "And my foot started to pound."

"Matt," you say over the portable, making eye contact with your partner through the thick safety glass of the control room. "I need you to bring that oxygen down to me and hurry the nurse up."

ILLNESS-RELATED EMERGENCIES

People get sick all the time. Sometimes the illness is minor and lasts only for a short time, such as a cold or the common flu. Illnesses such as diabetes, epilepsy, or asthma can remain with people for a lifetime and be very difficult to manage day in and day out. If not managed well, some illnesses can evolve into life-threatening emergencies requiring immediate attention and in some cases more advanced care. One of the keys to successful management of an illness-related emergency is a thorough assessment of the ill person.

Common Signs and Symptoms of Illness

There are endless causes of illness. A person can become ill suddenly or experience a flare-up of an existing illness. It is not important that you immediately discover the reason for the illness in order to care for the person properly. Your assessment will be aimed at addressing and caring for any immediate life threats and then gathering as much information as possible about what the ill person is feeling so that you can share this information with the EMS team.

8.1 List the common signs and symptoms of a general illness.

Some of the more common signs of an illness include:

- Altered mental status (confusion)
- Unresponsiveness
- Abnormal pulse or breathing
- Abnormal skin signs
- Unusual breath odors
- Uncontrolled muscle activity

Some of the more common symptoms of an illness include:

- Chest or abdominal pain (▼ Figure 8.1)
- Dizziness or headache

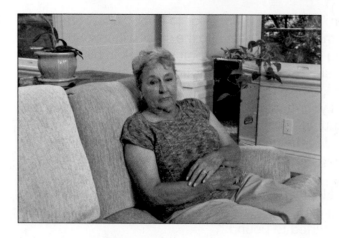

Figure 8.1 Abdominal pain is a common symptom of illness.

- Numbness or tingling
- Difficulty breathing
- Fever or chills
- Nausea
- Itching or burning skin

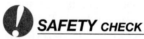

SAFETY CHECK

Always wear proper personal protective equipment such as gloves and a mask to minimize becoming exposed to an illness from someone you are caring for. ●

MAKE A NOTE

Illnesses are often referred to as "medical emergencies" and injuries are often referred to as "traumatic emergencies." ●

Assessment of the Ill Person

8.2 Explain the steps for assessing an ill person.

The care you provide to an ill person will depend on what you find during your assessment. The same steps for an assessment that were introduced in the last chapter are used with the person who is having a medical emergency:

- Scene size-up
- Primary assessment
- Secondary assessment
  - History
  - Physical examination
- Reassessment

Once you have determined that the scene is safe for you to enter, you will approach the ill person, introduce yourself, gain consent, and begin performing the primary assessment. If all is well with the primary assessment, you will continue on with the secondary assessment. You must not continue with the secondary assessment until all challenges related to airway, breathing, circulation (ABCs), and bleeding have been addressed.

The secondary assessment for ill persons almost always begins by obtaining the chief complaint. The chief complaint is what the person states is wrong with him. For instance, he might say, "I'm having trouble breathing," or "I get dizzy every time I try to sit up." Once you have determined the chief complaint, you can use the SAMPLE history tool that was introduced in the last chapter to further investigate the ill person's signs, symptoms, and medical history.

The other half of the secondary assessment is the physical exam. You will look at and perhaps feel any areas of complaint as appropriate. It is important to always let the person know exactly what you are doing and seek his permission to touch him or expose any parts of his body before doing so. The physical exam can be performed at the same time as or after the SAMPLE history. This will depend more on how much experience you have performing the assessment and your ability to multitask.

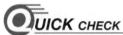

UICK CHECK

If there is a problem with the primary assessment, must you still do your best to complete a secondary assessment before EMS arrives? Why or why not? ●

CARING FOR SPECIFIC ILLNESSES

Altered Mental Status

A change in mental status is one of the most common signs that a person may be experiencing a sudden illness (▼ Figure 8.2). A normal mental status is one where the person is fully aware of who he is, where he is, what time it is, and what is going on around him. A lack of awareness in one or more of these areas is a sign of **altered mental status** and could be evidence of an underlying illness.

8.3 Explain the common causes of altered mental status.

altered mental status a change or decrease in mental abilities or responsiveness.

Figure 8.2 Common causes of an altered mental status.

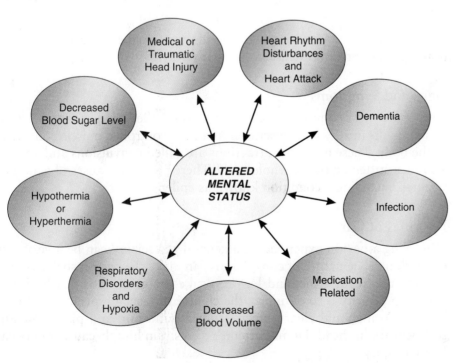

Signs and Symptoms

8.4 Describe the signs and symptoms of a person with an altered mental status.

Signs and symptoms of an altered mental status include:

- Decreased level of responsiveness (sleepy or sluggish)
- Confusion/disorientation
- Asking repeated questions
- Agitation or aggression

Priorities of Care

8.5 Explain the appropriate care for a person with an altered mental status.

The primary concern for a person with an altered mental status is an open and clear airway. As a person becomes less responsive, the ability to manage the airway adequately diminishes. You will need to closely monitor the person's airway and breathing status at all times.

Since the person with an altered mental status is likely going to be unable to provide you with much information about his chief complaint or medical history, you will need to rely on others at the scene for information. Gather as much information as you can from what you see at the scene, what you may know about the person, and what others tell you. This information may be helpful to the EMS team when they arrive.

If the person's ABCs are fine, and it is safe for you to do so, perform a physical exam, looking for any additional signs and symptoms related to the problem. Do not attempt to perform a physical exam if there are any problems with the ABCs. Management of the primary assessment is your top priority. If available, provide supplemental oxygen according to your protocols. Sometimes the most appropriate care is simply monitoring the ABCs, providing reassurance, and waiting for EMS providers to arrive.

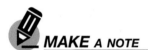

MAKE A NOTE

Anyone with an altered mental status should be considered seriously ill, and you should call 911 immediately. ●

Seizures

Seizures are caused by an interruption of the normal electrical activity in the brain and can present themselves in many ways.

Signs and Symptoms

8.6 Describe the signs and symptoms of a person experiencing a generalized seizure.

generalized seizure a common type of seizure that results in a loss of consciousness and uncontrolled muscle contractions of the body.

convulsions uncontrolled muscle contractions of the body.

epilepsy a condition affecting the brain and causes seizures.

One of the most common types of seizures is called the **generalized seizure**, which results in a loss of consciousness and uncontrolled muscle contractions of the body. These muscle contractions are called **convulsions** and appear as a sudden stiffening of the whole body. There are many causes of generalized seizures, including a condition known as **epilepsy**.

Priorities of Care

8.7 Explain the appropriate care for a person experiencing a generalized seizure.

Observing a person experiencing a generalized seizure can be a very frightening thing. The nature of convulsions can make the person shake violently, causing the head, arms, and legs to strike the ground or nearby objects. Your top priority is to minimize the chance that such a person could harm himself. You should clear objects from around him and place something soft beneath his head. Do not attempt to restrain him, because it may cause further injury.

It is not uncommon for a person experiencing a seizure to have a partial or complete airway obstruction. Noisy breathing is a sign of partial obstruction, which can be caused by soft tissues such as the tongue or an accumulation of saliva or blood. In rare cases, the airway can become completely obstructed during the seizure. There is no need to attempt to clear the airway in these cases, since the seizure is likely to last only a minute or so. Do not try to force the mouth open with any hard implement or with your fingers. A person having a seizure *cannot* swallow his tongue. Focus on protecting the person from injury and allow the seizure to run its course.

Once the seizure has ended and the convulsions have stopped, perform a primary assessment and confirm that the person is breathing adequately. In most cases, the person will begin breathing normally right away. He will remain unresponsive for several minutes as he slowly recovers from the seizure. This state is called the **postictal** state, which is quite normal.

postictal an unresponsive state of the body that follows a generalized seizure.

To assist in maintaining an open and clear airway, it is recommended that you place the person in the recovery position once the convulsions have stopped. It will be important to begin talking to the person even before he wakes, because often the person can hear what is going on around him even though he appears to be unconscious. Provide reassurance as he begins to wake up. If possible, attempt to get any medical history from bystanders or family members.

In most cases, a generalized seizure in someone who has epilepsy is not a medical emergency, even though it may look like one. A typical epileptic seizure will stop on its own after a minute or two without ill effects. The average person is able to continue about his business after a rest period and may need only limited assistance or no assistance at all.

A seizure can become an emergency when convulsions last more than five minutes or if a person has trouble breathing following a seizure. A person also can become injured during a seizure.

If you suspect that the person is having a seizure, activate your Emergency Action Plan or call 911.[1]

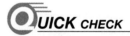

QUICK CHECK

Assuming that the scene is safe, what is your top priority when caring for a person who is actively convulsing from a seizure? ●

Brain Attack (Stroke)

A **brain attack (stroke)** occurs when blood flow to a portion of the brain is interrupted. This can be caused by either a rupture or a blockage of an artery that supplies blood to the brain. A brain attack can happen quite suddenly and without any warning, although many brain attack victims will experience a severe headache prior to an event.

brain attack (stroke) a condition caused by interruption of blood flow to a portion of the brain.

Signs and Symptoms

Signs and symptoms of a brain attack include:

- Sudden change in mental status (confused to unresponsive)
- Headache
- Vision problems
- Slurred speech

8.8 Describe the signs and symptoms of a person experiencing a stroke (brain attack).

[1]Epilepsy Foundation of America, *First Aid for Seizures* (Landover, MD: Epilepsy Foundation of America, n.d.), http://www.epilepsyfoundation.org/about/firstaid/index.cfm (accessed January 11, 2010).

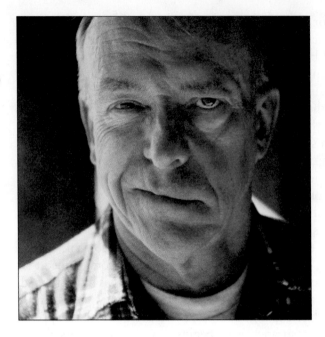

Figure 8.3 An abnormal drooping appearance on one side of the face may be a sign of a brain attack. (© Michal Heron Photography)

- Facial droop (▲ Figure 8.3)
- Paralysis of one side of the body

Priorities of Care

8.9 Explain the appropriate care for a person experiencing a stroke (brain attack).

As for anyone with an altered mental status, the priority of care is to ensure that the person has a good airway, adequate breathing, and adequate circulation (ABCs). You must constantly monitor the status of the airway and breathing, because it may be difficult for the person to manage his own airway and maintain adequate respirations. If you determine the person's breathing is not adequate (too slow or too shallow), you may need to provide rescue breaths.

Place the person in the recovery position. This will help in maintaining an open and clear airway. Understand that an unresponsive person may be able to understand you but unable to communicate in return. Continue to reassure the person and let him know exactly what you are doing at all times. Attempt to gather a SAMPLE history from bystanders or family members and pass this information on to the EMS team when they arrive. If supplemental oxygen is available, provide it according to your protocols.

Stroke treatment is time sensitive! Many stroke victims who get to the hospital emergency department quickly are less likely to have long-term impairment.

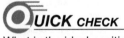 **CHECK**

What is the ideal position for anyone with an altered mental status who does not have a neck or back injury? ●

Diabetes

diabetes a condition that results when the body is unable to produce an adequate supply of insulin or when the body can no longer utilize insulin well.

Diabetes is a condition that results when the body is unable to produce an adequate supply of insulin or when the body can no longer utilize insulin appropriately. Insulin is necessary to ensure that the sugar the body takes in is properly distributed to all cells and used for energy. Too much or too little sugar can result in a diabetic emergency.

Normally, a diabetic person can manage his condition by carefully monitoring food intake and/or with medication. Every so often circumstances are such that an imbalance occurs, resulting in a diabetic emergency. If left untreated, a diabetic emergency can result in coma and even death.

Signs and Symptoms

Signs and symptoms of a diabetic emergency include:

- Altered mental status (confused or disoriented)
- Pale, moist skin
- Irritable or unusual behavior
- Fruity or sweet smell on the breath
- Unresponsiveness

8.10 Describe the signs and symptoms of a person experiencing a diabetic emergency.

A good SAMPLE history should include questions related to the person's medical history. It is appropriate to ask the person or bystanders if the person is diabetic. If so, asking when he last ate and if and when he may have taken his medication will help define the type of emergency that is occurring. It is not necessary for you to determine the exact cause of the emergency because Emergency Responder care will be the same no matter the cause.

Priorities of Care

Once again, your first priority will be to perform a thorough primary assessment and ensure adequate ABCs. If the person is semi-responsive to unresponsive, place him in the recovery position and monitor the ABCs until the EMS team arrives.

8.11 Explain the appropriate care for a person experiencing a diabetic emergency.

If the person is responsive and he can swallow without difficulty, it is appropriate to have him eat or drink something with sugar in it. A regular (non-diet) soda, orange juice, or sugar water are all appropriate. Instruct the person to hold the cup or can and take small sips to help prevent choking. If all you have is something solid, such as a candy bar or some other type of food, make sure the person takes small bites and chews them thoroughly. Have him swallow each sip or bite completely before offering another.

Depending on the cause of the diabetic emergency, you may see the person begin to feel better within a few minutes of taking in the sugar. Even so, you should still activate 911 and insist that he be evaluated by the EMS team or someone with more advanced training. If available, provide supplemental oxygen according to your protocols.

Chest Pain

Chest pain is the most common symptom of a heart attack and should be taken very seriously. A **heart attack** occurs when blood flow to the heart muscle is interrupted enough to cause muscle damage resulting in chest pain. In the worst-case scenario, the damage to the heart muscle is significant enough to cause cardiac arrest. Cardiac arrest occurs when the heart stops pumping blood.

It is possible to have chest pain related to the heart without having an actual heart attack. This pain is called **angina**, which is caused by an inadequate supply of blood to the heart muscle. Even though angina does not cause any actual heart muscle damage, it is a serious symptom of a heart problem and should be cared for just like a heart attack.

heart attack a condition that occurs when blood flow to the heart muscle is interrupted enough to cause muscle damage.

angina chest pain caused by an inadequate supply of blood to the heart muscle.

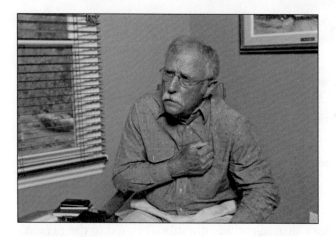

Signs and Symptoms

8.12 Describe the signs and symptoms of a person experiencing chest pain.

Signs and symptoms of a heart problem include:

- Chest pain (▲ Figure 8.4)
- Pressure/heaviness in the chest
- Radiating pain (arms, neck, back)
- Pale, moist skin
- Sweating
- Shortness of breath

MAKE A NOTE

The most common symptom of heart attack in both men and women is chest pain or discomfort. However, symptoms may also include discomfort in other areas of the upper body, shortness of breath, sweating, nausea, vomiting, and dizziness.[2]

Priorities of Care

8.13 Explain the appropriate care for a person experiencing chest pain.

If in doubt, care for all chest pain as though it were a heart attack. You have no way of knowing for certain what is going on with the person, so you must provide care based on the worst-case scenario. If you think the person is having a heart attack, activate your Emergency Action Plan or call 911 immediately. Taking aspirin during a heart attack can be life-saving. If the person is awake and alert, is not exhibiting signs or symptoms of a stroke, and does not have an allergy to aspirin, he or she should be encouraged to chew one adult or two low-dose "baby" aspirin while waiting for EMS to arrive.

Provide lots of reassurance and keep the person at rest and in a comfortable position. In most cases, he will prefer sitting up rather than lying down. Use the SAMPLE assessment tool to gather as much history about the situation as possible. If available, provide supplemental oxygen according to your protocols.

[2]O'Connor RE, Brady W, Brooks SC, Diercks D, Egan J, Ghaemmaghami C, Menon V, O'Neil BJ, Travers AH, Yannopoulos D. Part 10: acute coronary syndromes: 2010 American Heart Association Guidelines for Cardiopulmonary Resuscitation and Emergency Cardiovascular Care. *Circulation.* 2010;122(suppl 3):S787–S817.

Breathing Problems

A sudden onset of difficulty breathing is one of the most common emergencies an Emergency Responder will see. There are many causes of difficulty breathing, including asthma, allergic reaction, heart attack, and anxiety. Difficulty breathing can range from a very mild shortness of breath to a feeling that one cannot breathe at all. This is one of the scariest emergencies that anyone can experience. As an Emergency Responder, you will need to be able to control not only your fear but also the fear of the person experiencing the emergency. Helping him control panic is a key to helping him cope with the emergency.

Signs and Symptoms

Signs and symptoms of difficulty breathing include:

- Labored breathing
- Increased breathing rate
- Noisy breathing
- Anxiety
- Use of accessory muscles
- Cyanosis (bluish color of the lips and nail beds)

8.14 Describe the signs and symptoms of a person experiencing difficulty breathing.

When breathing becomes difficult, it becomes more obvious. In most cases, if the breathing difficulty is moderate to severe, it will be obvious as you approach the person. It is common for the person to assume a position with hands on the knees and shoulders held high. This is called the **tripod position** and can be performed either sitting or standing (▼ Figure 8.5). This

tripod position a position in which a person who is having difficulty breathing will get into so it is easier to breathe; the hands are on the knees and shoulders are held high.

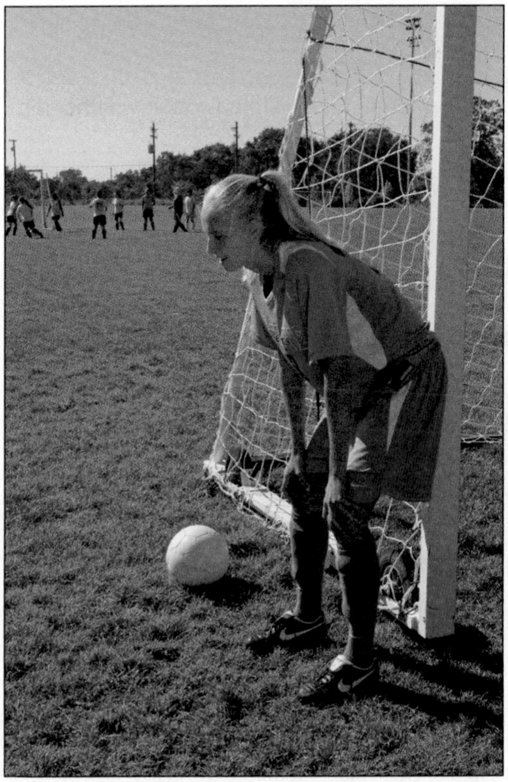

Figure 8.5 The tripod position helps the person move air in and out of the lungs.

cyanosis bluish color of the lips and nail beds.

position makes it easier to move air in and out of the lungs. In severe cases you might see a bluish color to the person's lips and nail beds. This is called **cyanosis** and is a sign of inadequate oxygen supply to the tissues.

Priorities of Care

8.15 Explain the appropriate care for a person experiencing difficulty breathing.

Initial care of the person with difficulty breathing should be focused on trying to calm him down and getting him to breathe more normally. This is easier said than done, but it must be attempted. Activate your Emergency Care Plan or call 911 sooner rather than later, because a breathing emergency can progress very rapidly. You do not want to delay care!

Allow the person to maintain the position that is most comfortable for his condition. Use the SAMPLE assessment tool to gather as much history as possible. You will want to determine if he has any existing respiratory problems and if he has been prescribed medication for such an event. The most common type of medication for breathing problems is a metered-dose inhaler (▼ Figure 8.6). You may assist the person in using the inhaler by handing it to him and encouraging him to use it as prescribed. First check to see that the medication is indeed prescribed to the person and that it has not expired. Instruct the person to use it just as the doctor recommended. If the victim is unable to administer his prescribed medication without assistance, the Emergency Responder should help to administer it.[3] Do not assist with the administration of expired medications.

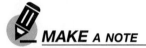

MAKE *A* **NOTE**

Never attribute difficulty breathing simply to anxiety. Never have a person with difficulty breathing breathe into a paper bag. If he does not have sufficient oxygen in his blood, this action could be fatal. Instead, apply oxygen and continue your attempts to calm him. ●

If breathing becomes so labored that the person can no longer breathe adequately, you may have to assist by giving him rescue breaths. If available, provide supplemental oxygen according to your protocols.

Follow the directions provided by your instructor or your Medical Director.

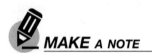

MAKE *A* **NOTE**

State laws, regulations, and occupational licensing requirements may prescribe specific practices, rules, standards, and other conditions for assisting with prescribed medications. ●

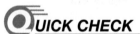

QUICK CHECK

Is it appropriate to encourage a person to take his medication whether it has expired or not? ●

Figure 8.6 A metered-dose inhaler.

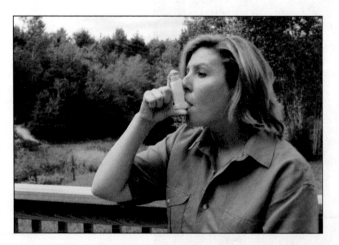

---

[3]Markenson D, Ferguson JD, Chameides L, Cassan P, Chung K-L, Epstein J, Gonzales L, Herrington RA, Pellegrino JL, Ratcliff N, Singer A. Part 17: first aid: 2010 American Heart Association and American Red Cross Guidelines for First Aid. *Circulation.* 2010;122(suppl 3): S934 –S946.

Cold-Related Emergencies

Overexposure to cold temperatures can lead to a generalized cooling of the body, resulting in a condition known as **hypothermia**. If left untreated, hypothermia can lead to a disruption in the normal function of the heart, which could lead to cardiac arrest and death. When specific areas of the body, such as the fingers, toes, and nose, get overexposed to very cold temperatures, frostbite can occur. **Frostbite** occurs when the tissues of the skin become frozen.

Signs and Symptoms

Signs and symptoms of cold exposure include:

Generalized hypothermia (▼ Figure 8.7):

- Cool skin temperature
- Shivering
- Altered mental state (confusion/disorientation)
- Loss of coordination

hypothermia a generalized cooling of the body's core temperature.

frostbite a condition that occurs when the tissues of the skin become frozen.

8.16 Describe the signs and symptoms of a cold-related emergency.

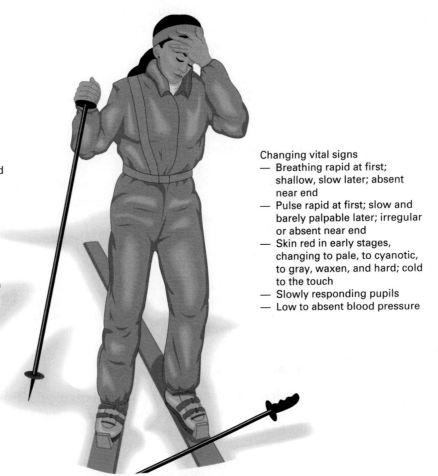

Decreasing mental status
— Amnesia, memory lapses, and incoherence
— Mood changes
— Impaired judgment
— Reduced ability to communicate
— Dizziness
— Vague, slow, slurred, or thick speech
— Drowsiness progressing even to unresponsiveness

Decreasing motor and sensory function
— Stiffness, rigidity
— Lack of coordination
— Exhaustion
— Shivering at first, little or no shivering later
— Loss of sensation

Changing vital signs
— Breathing rapid at first; shallow, slow later; absent near end
— Pulse rapid at first; slow and barely palpable later; irregular or absent near end
— Skin red in early stages, changing to pale, to cyanotic, to gray, waxen, and hard; cold to the touch
— Slowly responding pupils
— Low to absent blood pressure

Figure 8.7 Additional signs and symptoms of hypothermia.

Frostbite:

- Cool to cold skin
- Pale skin color
- Firm tissue
- Loss of sensation in the affected area

Priorities of Care

8.17 Explain the appropriate care for a person experiencing a cold-related emergency.

Once you have completed your primary assessment and ensured that the ABCs are okay, your next priority is to protect the person from additional heat loss. In most cases, your first step will be to remove him from the cold environment. Remove wet clothing, dry the skin if necessary, and cover him completely with warm blankets or similar material. Handle the person very gently, and do not give him anything to eat or drink. Seek more advanced care immediately, and do not allow the person to exert himself. If the patient is far from advanced care, provide active rewarming by placing the patient near a heat source or by placing heat packs or containers of warm, not hot, water in contact with the patient's skin. Chemical warmers should not be placed directly on frostbitten tissue because they can reach temperatures that can cause burns.

In cases of frostbite where EMS or medical attention is readily available, first move the victim to a warmer place and then remove any constricting jewelry and wet clothing. Place a sterile dressing between frostbitten fingers and toes, and wrap the frostbitten area with sterile dressings. Do not actively re-warm the affected area. Be sure to comfort, calm, and reassure the injured person during care.

If EMS or medical attention is *not* readily available, then immerse the frostbitten area/areas in warm water (not hot) for 20 to 30 minutes. The recommended water temperature is 98.6°F to 104°F (37°C to 40°C),[4] so check often and maintain the water temperature. Severe burning pain, swelling, and color changes may occur.

Do not re-warm the frostbitten body part if there is any chance that refreezing may occur. Do not rub or massage the affected area or disturb blisters on frostbitten skin. Do not give alcoholic beverages to a person suffering from hypothermia.

 SAFETY CHECK
_____

You must be prepared for the environment that you will be working in. As an Emergency Responder, you are just as susceptible to the exposure to heat and cold as the person you are caring for. ●

Heat-Related Emergencies

heat stroke a condition that occurs when the normal cooling mechanisms of the body are unable to keep the body cool.

Much like exposure to cold can lead to cold-related emergencies, overexposure to a hot environment can lead to heat-related emergencies. The most severe of the heat-related emergencies is called **heat stroke**. Heat stroke occurs when the

_____

[4]Markenson D, Ferguson JD, Chameides L, Cassan P, Chung K-L, Epstein J, Gonzales L, Herrington RA, Pellegrino JL, Ratcliff N, Singer A. Part 17: first aid: 2010 American Heart Association and American Red Cross Guidelines for First Aid. *Circulation.* 2010;122(suppl 3):S934–S946.

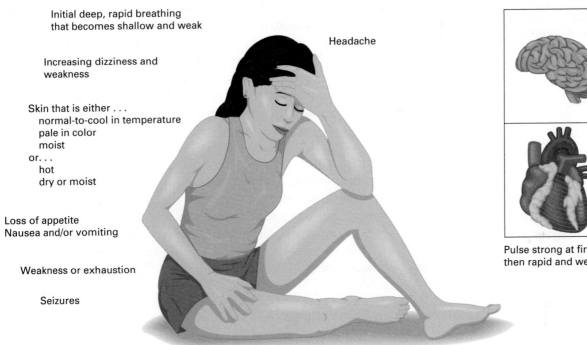

Altered mental status, possible unresponsiveness

Initial deep, rapid breathing that becomes shallow and weak

Increasing dizziness and weakness

Headache

Skin that is either . . .
normal-to-cool in temperature
pale in color
moist
or. . .
hot
dry or moist

Loss of appetite
Nausea and/or vomiting

Weakness or exhaustion

Seizures

Muscle cramps

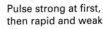

Pulse strong at first, then rapid and weak

Figure 8.8 Additional signs and symptoms of a heat-related emergency.

normal cooling mechanisms of the body, such as sweating, are unable to keep the body cool, allowing the body temperature to rise in excess of 105°F. Heat stroke is a true, life-threatening medical emergency that quickly can cause permanent damage to the organs, including the brain and spinal cord.

Signs and Symptoms

Signs and symptoms of a heat-related emergency include: (▲ Figure 8.8)

- Altered mental status
- Hot, moist or dry skin
- Weakness or exhaustion
- Muscle cramps
- Dizziness

8.18 Describe the signs and symptoms of a person experiencing a heat-related emergency.

In heat stroke, the overheating of the brain causes the altered mental status and can be a life-threatening emergency. A less severe type of heat emergency is called **heat exhaustion** and often presents before heat stroke. The most notable difference between heat exhaustion and heat stroke is an altered mental status.

heat exhaustion a condition marked by dizziness, nausea, and weakness and caused by overheating of the body.

🧒 *PEDIATRIC CARE*

Children are often unable to put on or remove their own clothing when confronted with extremes of temperature. For this reason, they are more vulnerable than the typical adult patient. ●

Priorities of Care

8.19 Explain the appropriate care for a person experiencing a heat-related emergency.

The priorities of care for a heat-related emergency will depend somewhat on the responsiveness of the person. If he has an altered mental status, you must first ensure that the ABCs are okay. Once completed, your next priority will be to cool the person as quickly as possible. Step one would be to get him to a cooler environment, if possible. This can be accomplished by moving him to a shady area or shielding him from direct sunlight. If possible, you also may move him into an air-conditioned environment.

For heat exhaustion, you can have the person lie down and then you can apply cool towels or cold packs to the arm pits, neck, and abdomen. Be careful not to overcool the person.

If you suspect heat stroke, begin aggressive cooling. Spray or pour water on the victim and fan him. Apply ice packs to the victim's neck, groin, and armpits and/or cover the victim with a wet sheet.

If the person is unresponsive, place him in the recovery position to protect the airway, and then continue to provide cooling until the EMS providers take over emergency care.

QUICK CHECK

Heat stroke is a life-threatening condition. What is your priority of care? ●

Poisoning and Overdose

Any substance that is harmful to the body is referred to as a poison. Poisons can enter the body in one of four ways:

- Ingestion (swallowing)
- Injection (bite or sting)
- Absorption (through the skin)
- Inhalation (breathing in)

 PEDIATRIC CARE

Children are very vulnerable to accidental overdose and poisoning. Call 911 or the Poison Control number for guidance before providing any care. ●

The most common type of poisoning occurs by ingestion and usually involves small children.

An **overdose** occurs when a person ingests too much of a substance such as a medication. While the medication in normal doses is a good thing, too much medication can become toxic and act like a poison to the body. Overdoses can occur on purpose or by accident.

overdose occurs when a person ingests too much of a substance such as a medication.

Signs and Symptoms

8.20 Describe the signs and symptoms of a person experiencing an overdose or poisoning.

Common signs and symptoms of a poisoning or overdose include:

- Altered mental status
- Convulsions
- Difficulty breathing
- Shallow respirations
- Burns around the mouth

Priorities of Care

The signs and symptoms of a poisoning or overdose vary widely depending on the substance involved. For this reason, your initial priority once again will be to ensure that the ABCs are okay. In a worst-case scenario, the person's breathing will be slow and shallow. If this occurs, you must provide rescue breaths.

Once you have addressed any issues related to the primary assessment, you then will focus on obtaining as much history as you can regarding what the person may have ingested, when he ingested it, and in what quantity.

For swallowed poison, call the National Poison Help Number at 1-800-222-1222 to talk to a poison expert. Follow the treatment recommendations given. Do not induce vomiting or give water, milk, activated charcoal, or syrup of ipecac to the victim unless you are advised to do so by Poison Control. Have all medicine bottles, containers, or samples of the poisoning substance available for EMS. If you think the substance may be dangerous to you or others, inform the EMS operators.

For skin contact with a poison, quickly remove the victim's contaminated clothing. Rinse the skin with large amounts of tap water, and contact Poison Control or alert EMS.

For inhaled poison, make sure it is safe to help the victim. If so, get him to fresh air right away. Alert EMS.

If the person is unresponsive but the ABCs are okay, it is appropriate to place him in the recovery position. Many poisons can cause nausea and vomiting. Placing the person in the recovery position will decrease the likelihood that he will choke on his vomit. If available, provide supplemental oxygen according to your protocols.

Bites and Stings

The environment in which we all live contains many threats to our well-being. One of these threats is exposure to bites and stings from a variety of sources, such as snakes, spiders, and other insects. In most instances, the body will react in an attempt to fight off the poison that enters it. This reaction can sometimes be severe and cause a life-threatening illness.

 PEDIATRIC CARE

Due to the small size of a child's airway, it may swell and become obstructed much more quickly than an adult airway. Do not delay calling 911 for any child you suspect may be experiencing a severe allergic reaction. ●

Signs and Symptoms

Common signs and symptoms of a bite or sting include:

- Noticeable sting or bite marks on the skin
- Itching of the skin
- Difficulty breathing
- Altered mental status
- Hives
- Dizziness
- Nausea and vomiting

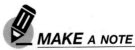 **MAKE** A **NOTE**

Providing rescue breaths for a person who has inhaled toxic fumes may be risky. If possible, utilize a barrier device with a one-way valve to prevent the possibility of breathing in toxic air from the ill or injured person. ●

8.21 Explain the appropriate care for a person experiencing an overdose or poisoning.

8.22 Describe the signs and symptoms of emergencies related to bites and stings.

Priorities of Care

8.23 Explain the appropriate care for a person experiencing an emergency related to a bite or sting.

The care for a person who has been bitten or stung will depend somewhat on his signs and symptoms. He may have only a local reaction, which will include swelling or redness at the site. If he experiences more serious symptoms, such as difficulty breathing or altered mental status, you must activate your Emergency Action Plan and call 911.

Keep the person comfortable, and monitor the airway and breathing closely. If he feels dizzy or lightheaded, place him in the recovery position. If the bite or sting occurred to an arm or leg, it may be helpful to elevate the limb to slow the rate of absorption. Applying cool packs to the site also may aid in slowing the absorption of the venom. If his breathing becomes inadequate, you may have to assist by providing rescue breaths.

Bites from humans and animals should be flushed with large amounts of water. This will help clean the wound and minimize the chance of infection.

Snakebites

For snakebites to the arm or leg, immobilize the limb and elevate while waiting for EMS.

Jellyfish Stings

To inactivate the venom from jellyfish stings, the area affected should be liberally washed with vinegar as soon as practical. If vinegar is not available, a solution of baking soda and water may be used. For the treatment of pain, once the stingers are removed or deactivated, immerse the stings in hot water or have the patient take a hot shower. Use a temperature as hot as can be tolerated by the patient or approximately 45°C.

Severe Allergic Reaction

Severe allergic reaction, or anaphylaxis, is a sudden, severe allergic reaction that involves the whole body. In anaphylaxis, swelling of the throat and tongue can block the victim's airway, which is fatal without prompt treatment. It is critical for anyone with a history of anaphylaxis to keep epinephrine auto-injectors on hand at all times, because waiting for paramedics to arrive on scene could significantly increase the risk of death.

Signs and Symptoms

Signs and symptoms include the rapid onset of any of the following:

- Swelling of lips, eyelids, throat, and tongue
- Extreme difficulty breathing
- Coughing/wheezing
- Altered mental status
- Anxiety
- Hives/itching
- Nausea/vomiting

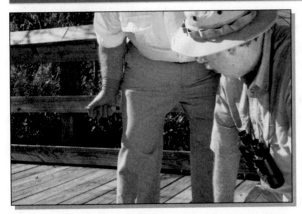

8.1.1 The Emergency Responder shows the patient how to hold the device.

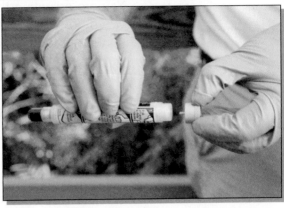

8.1.2 The Emergency Responder removes the safety cap.

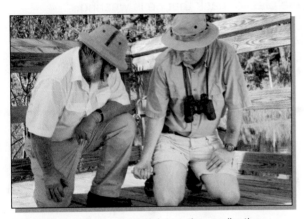

8.1.3 The person self administers the medication.

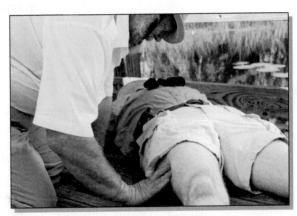

8.1.4 The Emergency Responder massages the injection site.

- Abdominal pain/cramping
- Diarrhea

Priorities of Care

The care for a person who is having a severe allergic reaction begins with assessing the ABCs. If the person carries a life-saving epinephrine auto-injector prescribed to him by a physician, help him use it (Scan 8.1). If he is unable to self-administer the medication, administer it to him yourself. Comfort, calm, and reassure the person while waiting for EMS providers to arrive.

Note that the beneficial effects of epinephrine may be limited to a short time, so seek immediate medical attention for the person. Make sure the used auto-injector box is sent to the emergency department with the person.

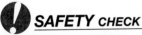 **SAFETY** *CHECK*
_____

Be alert when caring for persons who have been bitten or stung. You may be at risk for a sting or bite yourself. ●

THE HANDOFF

You are adjusting the nonrebreather mask on the confused inmate when two more correctional officers and a nurse in a medium-length white lab coat enter the day room from a loud door at the south end.

"Wow, Hector," the nurse says, looking at his face. "You definitely have something going on, don't you?"

The inmate nods and says, "Yes, ma'am."

"It's okay," she says, placing two fingers on his radial pulse. "We'll get you taken care of."

As the nurse is checking the inmate's pulse, she turns to one of the officers who came in with her and says, "Get an ambulance on the way. Tell them we have a 53-year-old male with a possible CVA."

"Hector, I'm thinking that you may have had a brain attack," she says, turning back to him and tapping the side of her own head. "When did you start having the pain that you told this officer about? Do you know?"

Hector blinks for a moment and then shakes his head, causing the oxygen to hiss from around the plastic mask that he is wearing.

"That's fine, that's fine," she says, patting his arm before turning to you. "Wonderful job recognizing the problem and getting oxygen on him. That's the best thing that you could've done."

CHAPTER REVIEW

Chapter Summary

- The assessment of an ill person should concentrate on the person's chief complaint.

- Common signs and symptoms of a general illness include altered mental status, difficulty breathing, chest or abdominal pain, and nausea.

- Some of the common causes of an altered mental status are such things as illness, brain attack, seizures, overdose, and allergic reactions.

- A person with an altered mental status may present as confused, sluggish, sleepy, or agitated.

- The signs and symptoms of a person experiencing a generalized seizure include a loss of consciousness and convulsions.

- The appropriate care for a person experiencing a generalized seizure should be focused on keeping the person from injuring himself. Once the seizure has ended, the priority is then to focus on the ABCs.

- The signs and symptoms of a person experiencing a stroke (brain attack) include an altered mental status, headache, slurred speech, and paralysis of one side of the body.

- The signs and symptoms of a person experiencing a diabetic emergency include an altered mental status; pale, moist, or reddish skin; unusual behavior; and a sweet odor in the breath.

- The signs and symptoms of a person experiencing chest pain include a pressure or heaviness in the chest; pain in the shoulders or arms; pale, moist skin; and shortness of breath.

- The signs and symptoms of a person experiencing difficulty breathing include labored breathing, increased rate, anxiety, and use of accessory muscles to breathe.

- The signs and symptoms of a cold-related emergency include cool skin temperature, shivering, altered mental status, and loss of coordination.

- Care for a person experiencing a cold-related emergency should include removing him from the cold environment as well as removing any wet clothing. Cover the person with warm blankets and do not give anything by mouth.

- The signs and symptoms of a person experiencing a heat-related emergency include altered mental status; hot, moist or dry skin; weakness; or exhaustion and muscle cramps.

- The appropriate care for a person experiencing a heat-related emergency should include moving him to a cool environment, having him lie down, and attempting to cool him with cold packs. If you suspect heat stroke, begin aggressive cooling with any resources available.

- The signs and symptoms of emergencies related to bites and stings include noticeable sting or bite marks, itching and redness of the skin, altered mental status, and difficulty breathing.

- General guidelines for the care of a person with an illness include keeping him in a position of comfort, providing reassurance, monitoring the ABCs, and providing rescue breaths if appropriate. If available, provide supplemental oxygen according to your protocols.

Quick Quiz

1. You are called to assist a coworker who is complaining of itchy skin, dizziness, and difficulty breathing. You should suspect:
   a. generalized seizure.
   b. brain attack.
   c. bite or sting.
   d. diabetic emergency.

2. Which one of the following is the one of the most common signs or symptoms of sudden illness?
   a. Abdominal pain
   b. Fever or chills
   c. Headache
   d. Altered mental status

3. Which one of the following is the most severe type of heat-related emergency?
   a. Heat exhaustion
   b. Heat cramp
   c. Heat stroke
   d. Dehydration

4. Which one of the following is a hormone required to ensure that cells can properly utilize sugar for energy?
   a. Glucose
   b. Insulin
   c. Epinephrine
   d. Creatinine

5. A boy has been found after being lost overnight in a wilderness area. He is confused and shivering and has skin that is cool to the touch. What is your first priority for his care?
   a. Remove him from the cold environment.
   b. Dry and warm his skin.
   c. Stop him from shivering.
   d. Ensure airway, breathing, and circulation.

6. The bluish color of skin caused by a lack of oxygen to the tissues is called:
   a. cyanosis.
   b. hypoxia.
   c. perfusion.
   d. contusion.

7. When the normal electrical activity in the brain is interrupted, it can cause:
   a. angina.
   b. hypoperfusion.
   c. seizures.
   d. strokes.

8. Poison can enter the body in all of the following ways EXCEPT:
   a. ingestion.
   b. excretion.
   c. absorption.
   d. inhalation.

9. A person with an altered mental status; exhaustion; muscle cramps; and hot, dry skin is most likely suffering from which one of the following conditions?
   a. Hypothermia
   b. Cardiac emergency
   c. Generalized seizures
   d. Heat-related emergency

10. Which one of the following is your primary concern for a person with an altered mental status?
    a. Open airway
    b. Safe environment
    c. Complete medical history
    d. Adequate assessment

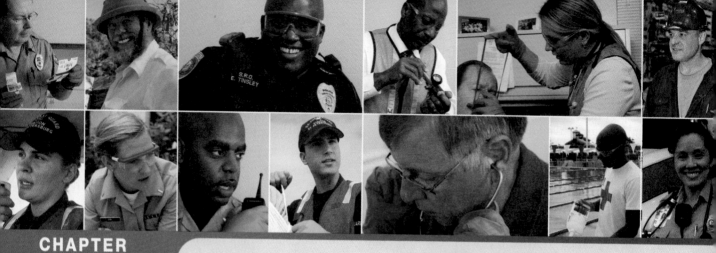

Caring for Soft-Tissue Injuries and Shock

KEY TERMS

The following terms are introduced in this chapter:

- amputation *(p. 120)*
- arteries *(p. 118)*
- bandage *(p. 121)*
- capillaries *(p. 118)*
- dressing *(p. 120)*
- evisceration *(p. 127)*
- hemostatic dressing *(p. 121)*
- occlusive dressing *(p. 121)*
- shock *(p. 119)*
- tourniquet *(p. 123)*
- veins *(p. 118)*

LEARNING OBJECTIVES

At the conclusion of this chapter and the associated instructor-guided lesson, the student will be able to:

Cognitive

9.1 Explain the importance of utilizing appropriate personal protective equipment (PPE) when caring for an ill or injured person with external bleeding. *(p. 118)*

9.2 Differentiate the characteristics of arterial, venous, and capillary bleeding. *(p. 118)*

9.3 Describe the signs and symptoms of shock. *(p. 119)*

9.4 List the common types of open wounds that result in external bleeding. *(p. 119)*

9.5 Explain the proper care for an injured person with active external bleeding. *(p. 120)*

9.6 State the purpose of a dressing. *(p. 120)*

9.7 State the purpose of a bandage. *(p. 121)*

9.8 State the purpose of a hemostatic agent. *(p. 121)*

9.9 Describe the signs and symptoms of internal bleeding. *(p. 123)*

9.10 Explain the proper care of an injured person with suspected internal bleeding. *(p. 126)*

9.11 Explain the proper care for an injured person with an impaled object. *(p. 126)*

9.12 Explain the proper care for a person with an open chest injury. *(p. 126)*

9.13 Explain the proper care for a person with an open abdominal injury. *(p. 127)*

9.14 Explain the proper care for an amputation injury. *(p. 128)*

9.15 Explain the proper care for nosebleed. *(p. 128)*

9.16 Explain the proper care for an injury to the eyes. *(p. 130)*

9.17 Differentiate superficial, partial-thickness, and full-thickness burns. *(p. 131)*

9.18 Explain the proper care for an injured person with a superficial, partial-thickness, and full-thickness burn. *(p. 131)*

Psychomotor

9.19 Demonstrate the proper techniques for controlling external bleeding.

9.20 Demonstrate the proper care for an injured person with suspected internal bleeding.

9.21 Demonstrate the proper care of an injured person with an open chest injury.

9.22 Demonstrate the proper care of an injured person with an open abdominal injury.

9.23 Demonstrate the proper care of an injured person with an impaled object.

9.24 Demonstrate the proper care of an injured person with an amputation injury.

9.25 Demonstrate the proper care of an injured person with a burn injury.

9.26 Demonstrate the proper care of an injured person with a dental injury.

Introduction

*I*NJURY is the leading cause of death in the United States for persons between the ages of one year and 40 years. Most of us will experience at least one significant injury of one kind or another in our lifetimes. This chapter describes the appropriate care for open wounds as well as the signs and symptoms for internal bleeding and shock.

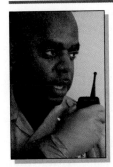

THE EMERGENCY

You work as a security guard at a local event arena and are standing backstage before the start of a rock concert. The lights slowly fade to black, leaving the large auditorium dark except for the occasional flicker of cell phone screens in the murmuring crowd. The band hurries past you to take their places on the darkened stage. As a single, growing tone from the keyboard vibrates through the building, you can sense the excitement of the audience even though you can't see anything.

Just as the electronic note reaches its crescendo—when you know the stage lights are about to explode into brilliant colors, illuminating the entire stage and beginning the show—you hear a loud crash on the dark stage followed by the din of cymbals and drums clattering to the floor.

"Help me!" a voice yells in the darkness.

"Come on, come on!" Erik, the band's tour manager, hits your shoulder as he runs past you.

You turn on your small flashlight, walk out onto the stage, and quickly find the band huddled around the drummer, who is trying to hold closed a large laceration on his right forearm. Blood jets from the gash in rhythmic explosions, spraying the haphazard drum kit and nearby stage with bright red splatters.

"Lights!" You hear the tour manager yelling toward the front of the stage. "Turn on the house lights!"

As the industrial lights high overhead pop on and slowly grow in brightness, thousands of faces suddenly come into view, and they are all watching you. You kneel next to the injured drummer and, using your gloved hands, put pressure on the open wound.

"Oh, man," the drummer says, lying back on the stage. "I'm really not feeling so hot."

"Erik," you say to the tour manager. "Call 911, now!"

BLEEDING AND SHOCK

Safety First!

9.1 Explain the importance of utilizing appropriate personal protective equipment when caring for an ill or injured person with external bleeding.

Injuries almost always result in damage to the soft tissues that make up the skin and muscles. Damage to soft tissues almost always results in bleeding. For this reason, take a moment now to review Chapter 3, where the importance of always utilizing appropriate personal protective equipment (PPE) whenever you are caring for an injured person is described. In addition to wearing protective gloves, remember to utilize eyewear. Prescription glasses, sunglasses, and special safety glasses are all appropriate for protecting your eyes against being splashed with blood or other body fluids.

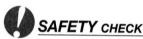 **SAFETY** CHECK

Be sure to don all appropriate personal protective equipment prior to approaching an injured person. When someone is bleeding, the risk of becoming exposed is high, but the risk can be managed easily with the proper protection. ●

Types of Bleeding

9.2 Differentiate the characteristics of arterial, venous, and capillary bleeding.

Blood is transported throughout the body in three types of vessels—arteries, veins, and capillaries.

arteries blood vessels that transport oxygen-rich blood under high pressure to the organs and cells of the body.

Arteries are vessels that transport oxygen-rich blood under high pressure to the organs and cells of the body. Arteries typically run deep within the body and close to bones for protection. Due to the pressure within, there is a significant potential for serious blood loss when arteries are damaged. Arterial blood is usually bright red in color and may be seen as spurting from the wound with each beat of the heart. Bleeding from arteries is also much more difficult to control than bleeding from other vessels due to the relative size of and higher pressure in the arteries.

veins vessels that transport blood depleted of oxygen under low pressure from the organs and cells and return it to the heart.

Veins transport blood that is depleted of oxygen under low pressure from the organs and cells and return it to the heart. Veins typically lie closer to the skin's surface and often can be seen as dark purple lines beneath the skin. The blood from veins is darker red in color and flows steadily from the vessel when damaged. Bleeding from veins often is easier to control due to the lower pressure inside the vessel.

capillaries the smallest of vessels that transport oxygenated blood.

Capillaries are the smallest of vessels that transport blood. The most common type of injury that damages the capillaries is a scrape or abrasion to the skin. Damage to capillaries typically causes bleeding that is bright red in color and oozes slowly from the wound.

Many soft-tissue injuries result in damage to one or more types of vessels, so bleeding may be coming from all sources at once, making it difficult to determine which type of vessel is damaged. Not to worry. You won't need to; your job will be to control any bleeding regardless of the type.

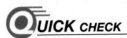
QUICK CHECK

Bleeding from which type of vessel is the most difficult to control? ●

Shock

Injuries that result in blood loss divert valuable blood from ever reaching the organs and cells. **Shock** results when the organs and cells of the body do not receive an adequate supply of well-oxygenated blood.

shock a condition that results when the organs and cells of the body do not receive an adequate supply of well oxygenated blood.

PEDIATRIC CARE

The smaller the person, the less blood volume he has to lose. What may appear to be minor bleeding for an adult could be life threatening for a child. Care for all bleeding in children as though it could be life threatening. ●

Signs and Symptoms

Injured persons who have lost a significant amount of blood will display signs and symptoms of shock, including:

9.3 Describe the signs and symptoms of shock.

- Pale, moist skin
- Altered mental status
- Increased heart rate
- Increased breathing rate
- Nausea and vomiting

Priorities of Care

Your priorities of care for a person who is displaying the signs and symptoms of shock should focus on maintaining the ABCs: Ensuring an open and clear airway, adequate breathing, and adequate circulation are key to the survival of this person. You also must assess for and immediately control any obvious bleeding.

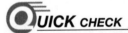
QUICK CHECK

What is it called when the organs and cells of the body do not receive an adequate supply of well-oxygenated blood? ●

OPEN WOUNDS

Any damage to the soft tissues of the body can result in bleeding. The most obvious type of bleeding is caused by open wounds, also known as external wounds. This occurs when the skin and underlying tissue become damaged due some type of external force.

9.4 List the common types of open wounds that result in external bleeding.

Types of Open Wounds

There are many types of open wounds, and each one has different characteristics depending on the mechanism of injury. Some of the more common types of open wounds include:

- **Superficial wound.** These are minor wounds that affect the outermost layers of skin and include minor cuts and scrapes.

- **Lacerations.** Often caused by sharp objects, lacerations will have straight and/or jagged edges.
- **Abrasions.** Often abrasions are caused by a forceful rubbing against a rough surface, such as the ground or pavement. Abrasions result when the outer layer of skin is damaged.
- **Avulsions.** Avulsions are caused by a tearing away of the skin or other soft tissue.
- **Penetrations.** These are caused by a sharp, pointed object or projectile such as a bullet.
- **Amputations.** An **amputation** occurs when a body part or limb is forcibly cut or torn from the body.

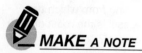

MAKE A NOTE

Do not let the unpleasant sight of open wounds distract you from your priorities of care. Always remember to manage the ABCs first! ●

amputation an injury that occurs when a body part or limb is forcibly cut or torn from the body.

 PEDIATRIC CARE

Aside from the pain, children can be very frightened by the sight of an open wound and the associated bleeding. Try to minimize the chances that the child may have to see his own wounds. ●

CARE FOR OPEN WOUNDS

9.5 Explain the proper care for an injured person with active external bleeding.

The first priority of care when dealing with open wounds is to control blood loss. Blood that is lost through open wounds can no longer circulate to the organs and cells, which can become starved for nutrition and oxygen. If the bleeding is not controlled, the injured person will suffer from shock and eventually die. This is why your care must focus on controlling the bleeding as soon as possible.

The first step in controlling bleeding is to apply direct pressure (Scan 9.1). It may be applied with a gloved hand, but it is preferred that you also use something clean and absorbent, such as a dressing or other absorbent material. Placing pressure directly over a wound "plugs the hole" and is successful in controlling most bleeding. Remember that bleeding from arteries will require more pressure and more time to control.

A dressing that becomes blood soaked beneath your hands indicates that the wound is still actively bleeding. If the first dressing becomes blood soaked, place additional dressings over the top of the first and continue to hold pressure. Do not remove the dressing that is directly over the wound because this may make the bleeding worse by removing any clots that have begun to form. It may be helpful to elevate the extremity. Be sure to confirm there are no injuries to the bones before attempting to elevate a limb. Your next step is to apply a tourniquet when major bleeding cannot be stopped by direct pressure and a pressure bandage. Tourniquets will be discussed in more detail later in this chapter.

9.6 State the purpose of a dressing.

dressing an absorbent pad typically made of gauze or similar material.

Dressings and Bandages

A **dressing** is an absorbent pad typically made of gauze or similar material. Dressings can be sterile or nonsterile and come in a variety of shapes and

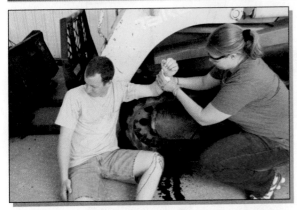

9.1.1 Hold direct pressure against the wound with an appropriate dressing.

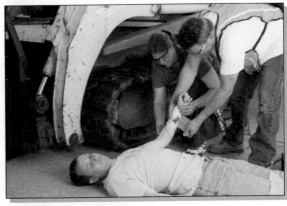

9.1.2 Apply and secure an elastic pressure bandage.

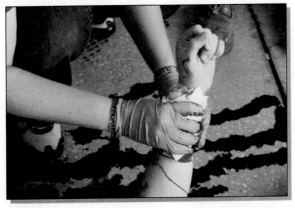

9.1.3 Apply additional dressings on top of pressure bandage, if bleeding continues. If direct pressure and pressure bandaging do not control bleeding, consider using a tourniquet.

sizes. When applied to an open wound, a dressing should extend beyond the wound on all sides.

An **occlusive dressing** is made of plastic or gauze saturated with petroleum jelly so that air will not pass through it. Occlusive dressings are used on very specific wounds, such as wounds to the neck and chest.

Recent developments in dressing design have resulted in a product called a **hemostatic dressing** (▼ Figure 9.1). Hemostatic dressings contain clotting agents that assist in the rapid development of blood clots at the opening of the wound, resulting in rapid control of bleeding.

The use of hemostatic agents, when standard methods fail to control life-threatening bleeding, is acceptable. More research is necessary to determine the best agent and conditions for use. Hemostatic agents are not currently in widespread first aid use at this time. Follow local protocol.

A **bandage** is made of cloth or gauzelike material that is designed to hold a dressing in place over a wound (▼ Figure 9.2). Bandages come in many shapes and sizes to accommodate a wide variety of applications.

occlusive dressing a dressing that does not allow air to pass through.

9.8 State the purpose of a hemostatic agent.

hemostatic dressing a dressing that contains clotting agents.

9.7 State the purpose of a bandage.

bandage a length of cloth or gauze-like material that is designed to hold a dressing in place over a wound.

Figure 9.1 Example packages of hemostatic dressings.

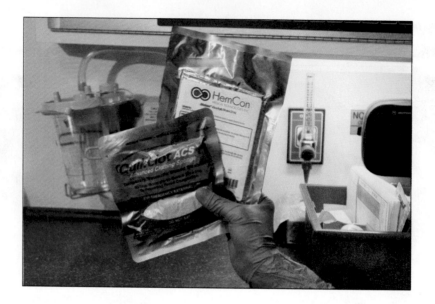

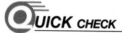

PEDIATRIC CARE

It is easy to wrap a bandage too tightly when your adrenaline is flowing. Just remember that a child will respond well to less pressure than necessary for an adult. ●

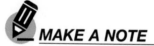

QUICK CHECK

What is the name of the device that is designed to be applied directly to a wound to assist with bleeding control? ●

MAKE A NOTE

Historically, the use of tourniquets was thought to be problematic. Recent research has shown that, when applied properly, they have proven to be effective tools for controlling severe bleeding. If you are NOT able to control bleeding within one to two minutes using direct pressure and elevation, apply a tourniquet. ●

Figure 9.2 A cravat can be used as a bandage to hold a dressing in place.

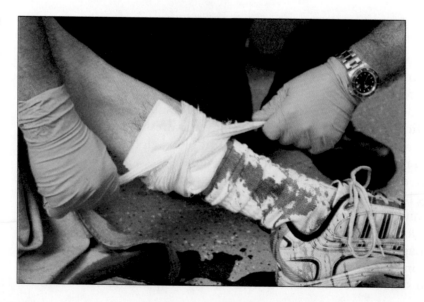

Application of a Tourniquet

A **tourniquet** is a device that when applied to a limb will stop all blood from flowing past. It can be improvised or purchased commercially and is designed to control bleeding from an arm or leg. Improvised tourniquets can be made of such things as a blood pressure cuff or a triangular bandage. Regardless of the type you use, the primary purpose of a tourniquet is to stop all blood flow from the wound site. Tourniquets should only be used by those who have received proper training in their use.

To apply a tourniquet using a triangular bandage, follow these steps (Scan 9.2 on page 124):

1. Fold a triangular bandage into a cravat approximately two inches wide.
2. Place the center of the cravat just above the wound site.
3. Wrap the cravat tightly around the limb, bringing both ends back to the top.
4. Tie a half knot over the top of the cravat and place a long, sturdy object such as a pencil or pen through the center of the knot.
5. Tie a full knot over the top of the device.
6. Twist the device until the bleeding at the wound site is controlled.
7. Document the time the tourniquet was applied and relay this information to the EMS responders.

In general, to apply a commercial tourniquet, you will follow these steps (Scan 9.3 on page 125):

1. While preparing the tourniquet, apply direct pressure over a thick dressing you have placed on the wound.
2. Apply the tourniquet proximal to the wound but not over a joint.
3. Tighten the tourniquet to the extent necessary to control bleeding.
4. Document the time the tourniquet was applied and relay this information to the EMS responders.

Do not remove or loosen the tourniquet once it is applied. Monitor the person's temperature and cover the person with a blanket if he becomes cold. If supplemental oxygen is available, provide it according to your protocols.

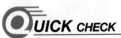

QUICK CHECK

Your attempts to control bleeding with direct pressure and elevation have failed. What should be your next step? ●

CLOSED WOUNDS

Wounds that occur inside the body are often called closed wounds and can result in bleeding inside the body. Closed wounds often are caused by strong forces against the body. Internal wounds are very difficult to detect and can quickly become life threatening.

tourniquet a device that when applied to a limb stops all blood flow past the device.

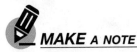

MAKE A NOTE

Tourniquets should only be used to control bleeding from an injured extremity such as an arm or leg. All other bleeding must be controlled using direct pressure. ●

9.9 Describe the signs and symptoms of internal bleeding.

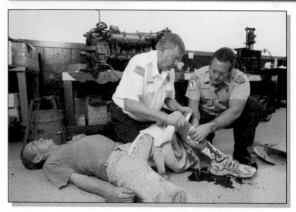

9.2.1 Fold a triangular bandage into a cravat approximately one to two inches wide.

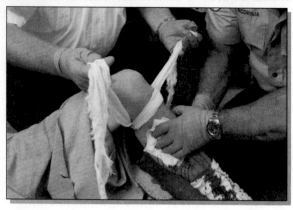

9.2.2 Place the center of the cravat just above the wound site.

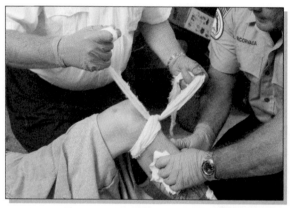

9.2.3 Wrap the cravat tightly around the limb, bringing both ends back to the top.

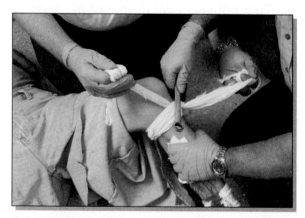

9.2.4 Tie a half knot over the top of the cravat, and place a long, sturdy object such as a pencil or pen through the center of the knot.

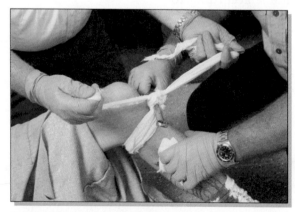

9.2.5 Tie a full knot over the top of the device.

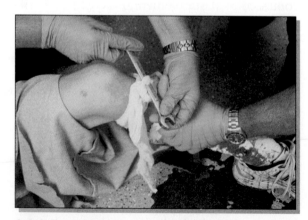

9.2.6 Twist the device until the bleeding at the wound site is controlled.

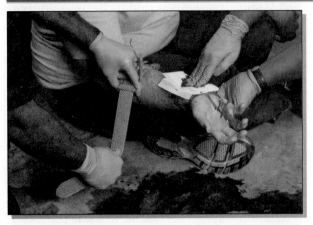

9.3.1 While preparing the tourniquet, apply direct pressure over the wound.

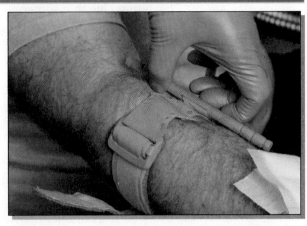

9.3.2 Apply the tourniquet proximal to (just above) the wound but not over a joint.

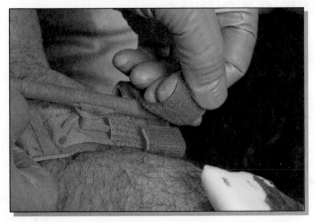

9.3.3 Twist the device to tighten the tourniquet to the extent necessary to control bleeding.

Internal Bleeding

One of the easiest ways to detect the possibility of internal bleeding is to assess the mechanism of injury. Any strong force against the body, especially in the areas of the chest, abdomen, and/or pelvis, has a high likelihood of causing internal injuries. Bruising is a sign of internal bleeding, but bruises may not show up for many hours after an injury has occurred.

It is best to care for any person who has suffered a significant injury to the body as if he has internal injuries and not wait for the signs and symptoms of shock to appear. Signs and symptoms of internal bleeding include:

- Pain
- Swelling
- Rigid or tight abdomen
- Bruising
- Difficulty breathing

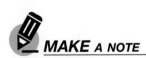

MAKE A NOTE

Internal bleeding is impossible to see or control without more advanced care. What you can do is identify the signs and symptoms and seek more advanced care as soon as possible.

While it is important to begin care for bleeding as soon as possible, it is often difficult to know that the person is bleeding internally. Sometimes your first clue that someone may be bleeding internally is that he begins to display the signs and symptoms of shock.

Whenever you suspect internal bleeding in an injured person, follow these steps:

1. Activate your Emergency Action Plan or call 911.
2. Monitor the ABCs.
3. Control any external bleeding.
4. Keep the person lying flat.
5. Monitor body temperature and cover the person with a blanket if he feels cold.
6. If available, provide supplemental oxygen according to local protocols.

CARING FOR SPECIFIC WOUNDS

Impaled Object

9.11 Explain the proper care for an injured person with an impaled object.

Sometimes an object can become impaled in a part of the body (▼ Figure 9.3). The object causes damage as it enters the body and can result in significant bleeding both internally and externally. In most instances it is recommended that you leave the object in place and attempt to stabilize the object to keep it from moving. There is a much greater risk for bleeding if the object is removed.

A time when it may be appropriate to remove an impaled object is when the object is interfering with your ability to maintain an open and clear airway, such as an object that has impaled the cheek.

Open Chest Injury

9.12 Explain the proper care for a person with an open chest injury.

Chest injuries can be life threatening because they can cause damage to internal organs such as the heart and lungs (▶ Figure 9.4). Especially dangerous

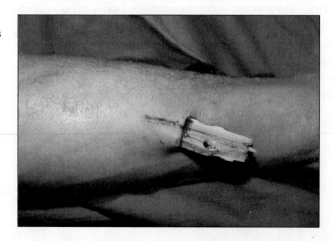

Figure 9.3 An impaled object in the forearm. (Charles Stewart, MD, and Associates)

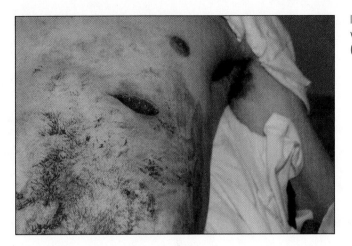

Figure 9.4 A gunshot wound to the chest. (© Edward T. Dickinson, MD)

are open wounds to the chest because of the possibility of air getting trapped inside. Your first priority is to control bleeding from any open wounds using direct pressure. If possible, you will want to cover an open chest wound with an occlusive dressing. An occlusive dressing will prevent air from being sucked into the chest through the wound, which causes dangerous pressure. An occlusive dressing can be made from something as simple as a piece of plastic or gauze saturated with petroleum jelly. Keep the person lying flat and as comfortable as possible.

Open Abdominal Injury

Open wounds to the abdomen can result in the exposure of the intestines (▼ Figure 9.5). This type of injury is called an **evisceration**. Your first priority will be to control any bleeding using direct pressure. Cover the wound with a large dressing that has been moistened with water, and carefully hold gentle pressure until bleeding is controlled. If water is not available, using a dry dressing is acceptable.

It will be important to keep the person lying flat and encourage him to be as still as possible. Any movement could make the wound worse.

9.13 Explain the proper care for a person with an open abdominal injury.

evisceration an open wound to the abdomen that results in the exposure of the intestines.

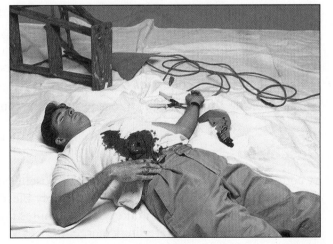

Figure 9.5 An open abdominal wound with an evisceration.

Figure 9.6 An amputation of the hand at the wrist. (Charles Stewart, MD, and Associates)

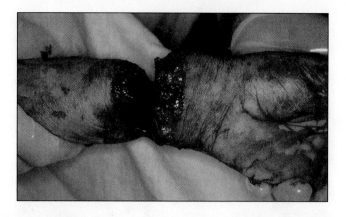

Amputation Injury

9.14 Explain the proper care for an amputation injury.

An amputation occurs when a part of the body such as a finger, hand, foot, or leg is separated from the body due to injury (▲ Figure 9.6). Bleeding from amputations can be anything from very mild to severe, depending on the mechanism that caused the injury.

Amputation injuries can be difficult for the Emergency Responder to manage due to their graphic nature. It is important that you not get distracted by the injury and forget to address the ABCs.

Your first priority will be to control any bleeding coming from the injury site. Do not worry about the amputated part until you have controlled the bleeding from the injury site. Your attempts to control bleeding should begin with direct pressure. Apply a tourniquet when major bleeding cannot be stopped by direct pressure and an elastic bandage.

Caring for the Amputated Part

Only after you have successfully controlled the injured person's bleeding will you then care for the amputated part. To care for an amputated part, follow these steps:

1. Cover the open wound with clean dressings.
2. Wrap the entire part in plastic. Small parts can be placed in a plastic bag.
3. Cool the amputated part by covering with a clean dressing and then placing it in a plastic bag. Place the bag in a mixture of ice and water or surround it with cool packs.
4. Be sure the amputated part goes with the person to the hospital.

QUICK CHECK

How should an amputated part be handled by the Emergency Responder? ●

Nosebleed

9.15 Explain the proper care for nosebleed.

A common type of bleeding wound is the nosebleed (▶ Figure 9.7). A nose can bleed following an injury, or it can simply bleed spontaneously without any injury at all. While it can take several minutes for a nose to stop bleeding, it is rarely ever a life-threatening emergency.

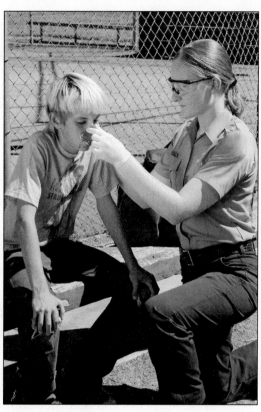

Figure 9.7 A common type of bleeding wound is a nosebleed.

To care for a person with a bloody nose, follow these steps:

1. Place a clean dressing over the nostrils while pinching the nostrils firmly, keeping them closed.

2. Have the person sit and lean forward as you continue to hold pressure on the nose.

3. Be patient. A nosebleed may take several minutes to control.

It is important to not let the person lean back, because this may direct blood toward the back of the throat and into the stomach. Blood in the stomach often will cause nausea and vomiting, and this will further complicate the situation. If blood does accumulate in the back of the throat, encourage the person to spit it out rather than swallow it.

 PEDIATRIC *CARE*

Nosebleeds are quite common in children and almost always are easy to manage. To help minimize the anxiety of the child at the sight of his own blood, use a dark towel or cloth, if possible, to help control the bleeding. ●

Dental Injuries

Injuries to the face and mouth often result in damage to the teeth. This can occur when the face and mouth are struck hard enough to cause teeth to break or become loose in their sockets. A tooth also can be knocked completely out of its socket if struck hard enough.

As always, once it is safe for you be begin caring for the injured person, your first concern should be for an open and clear airway. Broken teeth and

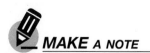 **MAKE** *A NOTE*

If you are unable to successfully control bleeding from a nosebleed in 15 minutes or less, consider seeking more advanced care. ●

blood can easily cause an obstruction of the airway. Have the person lean forward or place him in the recovery position to minimize any blood getting into the airway. Have him spit out any broken teeth.

If possible, place the teeth that have been knocked out in a cup of milk. If a source of milk is not readily available, wrap the teeth in clean gauze and make sure any broken teeth go with the person to the hospital or dentist.

If necessary, use clean gauze to apply gentle pressure to the open tooth socket to help control any bleeding.

Eye Injuries

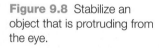

9.16 Explain the proper care for an injury to the eyes.

While rarely life threatening, injuries to the eyes can be devastating to the injured person. The eye is a hollow, fluid-filled globe made of delicate and very specialized tissue. Even the slightest injury can be both painful and debilitating. Your first priority will be to control any obvious bleeding with a clean dressing and gentle pressure. Do not attempt to remove any objects that may remain in the eye from the injury.

When caring for a person with eye injuries, follow these guidelines:

- Small foreign objects or debris on the surface of the eye can be flushed out with clean water or an eyewash solution.

- Injuries to the eye that are caused by a splashing of chemicals should be cared for by flushing the affected eye with large amounts of tap water. Position the person on their side with the affected eye downward and direct the flow of water from the inside edge of the eye. Be sure not to cause the fluid to get into the unaffected eye.

- Heat burns to the eyes should be cared for by placing moist dressings over both eyes.

If an object is protruding out of the eye, use dressings and bandages to stabilize the object (▼ Figure 9.8). Place several gauze pads around the object and secure them in place with a bandage. Whenever possible, cover both the affected eye and the unaffected eye. This will prevent movement of the protruding object, since both eyes move together.

It can be very frightening for the person with both eyes covered. Be sure to provide reassurance to minimize anxiety.

Figure 9.8 Stabilize an object that is protruding from the eye.

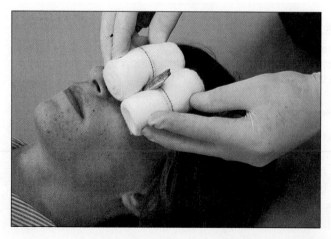

Children will be very frightened if you must cover both eyes due to an eye injury. Be sure to use lots of reassurance and tell the child everything that you are doing at all times. ●

Burn Injuries

Burns often are described by the mechanism that caused them and the severity of the burn. The three most common mechanisms of a burn injury are chemicals, electricity, and heat. (See Figure 9.9.)

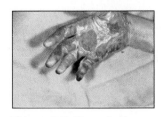

Figure 9.9 Burns to the hand may result in loss of function.

9.17 Differentiate superficial, partial-thickness, and full-thickness burns.

Classification of Burns

The severity of a burn is defined by the depth of the burn injury and the amount of surface area affected by the burn. There are three common descriptions for the depth of a burn:

- **Superficial.** These burns affect only the surface of the skin and cause a reddening of the skin with mild to moderate pain. The most common type of superficial burn is sunburn.
- **Partial thickness.** These burns affect the deeper layers of the skin and are characterized by blisters.
- **Full thickness.** These burns affect all layers of the skin and can reach the muscles and bones. Full-thickness burns are characterized by open charred skin.

In addition to the depth of the burn, the severity of a burn is determined by the amount of body surface area affected. The more surface area that is burned, the more severe the burn is.

Priorities of Care

First and foremost, you must make certain that it is safe for you to approach the injured person. Be careful not to become exposed to the same source that caused the person's burns. Once you have determined that it is safe to approach the person, extinguish all burning clothing. Remove any smoldering clothing as well, but be aware that the clothing may have melted to the skin. If there is resistance, leave the clothing in place.

9.18 Explain the proper care for an injured person with a superficial, partial-thickness, and full-thickness burns.

Immediately cool thermal burns with water that is room temperature. Cooling with water will help reduce pain, the depth of injury, and the need for skin grafting. Do not use ice or ice water because it can cause further injury to the burned tissues. Do not cool large burns as it may cause hypothermia, especially in children.[1] Monitor the person's ABCs carefully, because he may have difficulty breathing if he has inhaled hot air and/or smoke. If there is any indication that he may have inhaled hot smoke or air, call 911 immediately.

Never apply anything to an open or closed wound such as ointments, lotions, or butter. This will serve only to keep heat in. Do not break blisters.

---

[1]Markenson D, Ferguson JD, Chameides L, Cassan P, Chung K-L, Epstein JL, Gonzales L, Hazinski MF, Herrington RA, Pellegrino JL, Ratcliff N, Singer AJ; on behalf of the First Aid Chapter Collaborators. Part 13: first aid: 2010 American Heart Association and American Red Cross International Consensus on First Aid Science. *Circulation.* 2010;122(suppl 2):S582–S605.

If the burns are caused by chemicals, brush off any dry chemical prior to flushing with water. For burns caused by liquid chemicals, provide continuous flushing with large amounts of water for at least 15 to 20 minutes or until EMS arrives.

 PEDIATRIC CARE

What might appear at first glance to be a minor burn could be much more significant for a child. When in doubt, have all burns in children examined by an appropriate health-care provider. ●

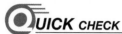UICK CHECK

What is the most appropriate method for caring for burns? ●

 SAFETY CHECK

Persons who have been burned often have been exposed to something that could still be a danger to the Emergency Responders. Approach the scene of a burn victim very cautiously, and be alert for any danger to you or others at the scene. ●

THE HANDOFF

The huge crowd remains strangely silent as you continue holding pressure on the drummer's tattooed forearm. The blood is no longer spurting, but it is dripping steadily between your gloved fingers.

With the clatter of equipment and hiss of portable radios, the stage is suddenly filled with firefighters, ambulance personnel, and stagehands. One of the EMTs kneels next to you and covers the injury with a large trauma dressing while the other EMT begins providing high-concentration oxygen with a nonrebreather mask.

You stand, blood dripping from your hands, and watch as the rescuers load the drummer onto the gurney and roll him quickly offstage. You look around and realize that you've never seen so much blood before, but you feel proud that you knew what to do and were able to help. You turn and walk off of the stage, trailed by the whistles and clapping of the crowd.

CHAPTER REVIEW

Chapter Summary

- Caring for bleeding wounds poses a greater risk of exposure to blood. Be sure to don proper personal protective equipment prior to approaching the injured person.

- Shock occurs when the organs and cells do not get an adequate supply of oxygen-rich blood. Signs and symptoms of shock include pale, moist skin; altered mental status; increased breathing and heart rates; and nausea and vomiting.

- Proper care for external bleeding includes applying direct pressure and a pressure bandage. Apply a tourniquet when major bleeding cannot be stopped using those methods. Monitor the ABCs and provide supplemental oxygen according to local protocols.

- The signs and symptoms of internal bleeding include pain, swelling, and a rigid abdomen. If internal bleeding is severe enough, the person also will display signs and have symptoms of shock.

- Care for suspected internal bleeding includes calling 911, keeping the person lying flat, monitoring the ABCs, and keeping him warm.

- The proper care for an injured person with an impaled object includes controlling any external bleeding and stabilizing the object. Do not remove impaled objects unless they interfere with managing the person's airway.

- The proper care for an open chest injury includes controlling external bleeding, applying an occlusive dressing, and monitoring the ABCs.

- The proper care for an open abdominal injury includes keeping the person lying flat, controlling external bleeding with direct pressure, and covering any exposed organs with a clean dressing.

- The proper care for an amputation injury includes controlling bleeding at the injury site and monitoring the ABCs. Care for the amputated part includes covering the amputated part with a clean dressing, wrapping in plastic, and keeping the part cool. Be sure to send the amputated part to the hospital along with the person.

- The proper care for a nosebleed includes using a clean dressing to firmly pinch the nostrils closed and having the person sit forward in a chair. Avoid allowing blood to flow back into the stomach.

- The proper care for a chemical eye injury includes flushing the eye with large amounts of water. For damage to an eye from injury, cover the eye gently with a clean dressing and then cover the unaffected eye to minimize movement of the injured eye.

- Burns can be caused by chemicals, electricity, and heat. The severity of a burn is classified by its depth—superficial, partial thickness, and full thickness—as well as how much of the body's surface is affected.

- Immediately cool thermal burns with water at room temperature. Do not use ice or ice water. Do not cool large burns.

Quick Quiz

1. You are caring for a woman with a scald burn from hot liquid. The skin of her forearm is red and blistered and she is in a lot of pain. You should:
   a. apply burn ointment.
   b. apply ice.
   c. Cool the burn with water.
   d. break the blisters.

2. As a member of your company's Emergency Response Team, you are called on the radio to assist with an evisceration injury. What is the single most important item to have to treat the injury?
   a. Sterile water
   b. A large dressing
   c. Cloth tape
   d. A plastic bag

3. What type of life-threatening trauma can be very difficult for Emergency Responders to detect?
   a. External bleeding
   b. Contusions
   c. Full-thickness burns
   d. Internal bleeding

4. When caring for open wounds, bandages are:
   a. placed directly against the wound to aid in clotting.
   b. rarely needed.
   c. used to hold dressings in place.
   d. usually replaced periodically.

5. Why is it important to bandage both eyes on a patient with an object protruding from only one eye?
   a. To prevent the patient from seeing the impaled object
   b. To keep the patient from moving the injured eye
   c. To protect the uninjured eye
   d. It is not necessary to bandage the uninjured eye.

6. You are assisting a bicycle crash patient who you suspect has internal bleeding. You should position the patient:
   a. lying flat on his back.
   b. on his side to keep his airway clear.
   c. sitting with his head between his knees.
   d. facedown with his head turned to the left.

7. When organs and cells are NOT getting an adequate supply of oxygen-rich blood, it is called:

   a. hyperperfusion.

   b. asphyxiation.

   c. hemostasis.

   d. shock.

8. Nosebleeds are best treated by pinching the patient's nostrils together and:

   a. having him tilt his head back.

   b. filling them with gauze.

   c. keeping his head in a neutral, in-line position

   d. having him lean forward in a chair.

9. Your patient has suffered an amputation of the right hand just above the wrist. Your first priority is to:

   a. keep the hand cool.

   b. control the bleeding.

   c. wrap the injured arm in plastic.

   d. apply pressure to the amputated hand.

10. When encountering open wounds that ooze bright red blood, you should suspect what type of bleeding?

    a. Arterial

    b. Venous

    c. Capillary

    d. Integumentary

11. Which one of the following injuries causes the tearing away of skin or soft tissues?

    a. Avulsion

    b. Laceration

    c. Contusion

    d. Amputation

12. Tourniquets are used to:

    a. slow blood loss from severe injuries.

    b. physically support injured extremities.

    c. stop all blood flow from a wound site.

    d. reduce pain by compressing damaged nerves.

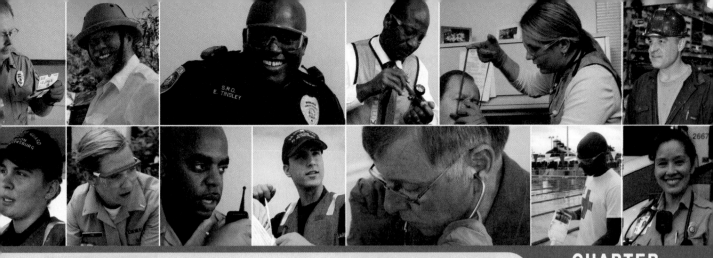

Caring for Muscle and Bone Injuries

LEARNING OBJECTIVES

At the conclusion of this chapter and the associated instructor-guided lesson, the student will be able to:

Cognitive

10.1 Identify the components that make up the musculoskeletal system. *(p. 136)*

10.2 Explain the functions of the musculoskeletal system. *(p. 136)*

10.3 List the four common types of musculoskeletal injuries. *(p. 138)*

10.4 Differentiate between an open and closed skeletal injury. *(p. 138)*

10.5 Describe the signs and symptoms of a musculoskeletal injury. *(p. 139)*

10.6 Explain the priority of care for an injured person with a suspected open skeletal injury. *(p. 140)*

10.7 Explain the importance of an appropriate assessment of the distal extremity. *(p. 141)*

10.8 Explain the appropriate care for an injured person with a skeletal injury. *(p. 142)*

Psychomotor

10.9 Demonstrate the appropriate assessment of a skeletal injury.

10.10 Demonstrate the appropriate care for a person with a long bone injury.

10.11 Demonstrate the appropriate care for a person with a joint injury.

10.12 Demonstrate the proper placement of an arm sling.

10.13 Demonstrate maintaining the hand/foot in the position of function during immobilization of an extremity.

KEY TERMS

The following terms are introduced in this chapter:

- angulation *(p. 140)*
- capillary refill *(p. 141)*
- closed fracture *(p. 138)*
- cravat *(p. 145)*
- dislocation *(p. 138)*
- ligaments *(p. 137)*
- manual stabilization *(p. 143)*
- open fracture *(p. 138)*
- position of function *(p. 143)*
- sling *(p. 145)*
- splint *(p. 143)*
- sprain *(p. 138)*
- strain *(p. 138)*
- swathe *(p. 145)*
- tendons *(p. 137)*

Introduction

*I*t is our muscles and bones that enable us to be mobile and active in our daily lives. Bones serve as the support structure for the body and provide the foundation for its basic shape. Muscles give us the ability to walk, run, and participate in day-to-day activities. Because the body can be so mobile, humans often put themselves at risk for injury.

Injury to muscles and bones are some of the most common emergencies that you will encounter as an Emergency Responder. This chapter describes some of the more common injuries and the steps to appropriately care for them.

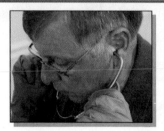

THE EMERGENCY

You are starting another year as a campus supervisor at the local high school, monitoring student interactions and keeping the hallways safe and moving. You are standing just east of the main entrance watching the talkative mass of students push through the doors and spill down the long, shining hallways into various classrooms.

"Hey!" You hear someone yell from outside. "That girl just fell down the stairs."

As the crowd of backpack-toting kids starts blocking the entrance, straining to see what happened, you push your way through.

"Come on, guys, get to class," you say, nearing the entrance. "Move it along. Don't block the doors."

The crowd around you starts moving, and you suddenly find yourself outside in the cool morning air, your breath rising in white clouds. At the foot of the steps leading to the school's main doors is a small crowd of students standing around a girl who is sitting on the pavement.

"Let me in," you say, gently moving students aside. "Go ahead and go to class."

When you reach the center of the dispersing group, you crouch down and ask the girl if she is okay. Her face is bright red and she blinks away tears, holding her left arm up. Her arm is deformed and already swollen halfway between the elbow and wrist. She lowers it back down and cradles it in her right arm.

"Did you hit anything else when you fell?" You ask, concerned about other injuries.

"No," she says through clenched teeth, fresh tears spilling down her cheeks. "I slipped and just sort of slid down the stairs and tried to stop myself at the bottom, and this happened to my arm."

"It's going to be okay. Just keep holding it steady like you are." You then grab your cellular phone and call 911.

10.1 Identify the components that make up the musculoskeletal system.

10.2 Explain the functions of the musculoskeletal system.

THE MUSCULOSKELETAL SYSTEM

The musculoskeletal system is really two separate systems that work in tandem with one another to allow us to move about. At the core is the skeletal system, which is made up of over 200 different bones (▶ Figure 10.1). The skeletal

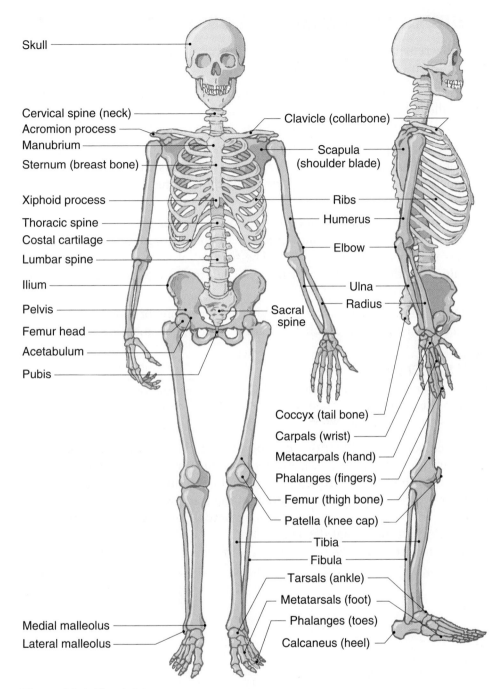

Skull

Cervical spine (neck)
Acromion process
Manubrium
Sternum (breast bone)

Xiphoid process
Thoracic spine
Costal cartilage
Lumbar spine

Ilium

Pelvis

Femur head
Acetabulum

Pubis

Clavicle (collarbone)

Scapula
(shoulder blade)

Ribs
Humerus
Elbow

Ulna
Radius

Sacral
spine

Coccyx (tail bone)
Carpals (wrist)
Metacarpals (hand)
Phalanges (fingers)
Femur (thigh bone)
Patella (knee cap)
Tibia
Fibula
Tarsals (ankle)
Metatarsals (foot)
Phalanges (toes)
Calcaneus (heel)

Medial malleolus
Lateral malleolus

Figure 10.1 The skeleton.

tendons the structures at the end of each muscle that attach directly to the bone.

ligaments tough, fiber-like tissues that connect two or more bones, typically at a joint.

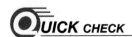**UICK** CHECK

Which structure holds two or more bones together at a joint? ●

system has several functions, including support, movement, protection, and cell production.

Overlaying the skeletal system is a complex system of muscles and other soft tissues, such as tendons and ligaments, that allow the body to walk, run, and move about with ease. **Tendons** are the structures at the end of each muscle that attach directly to the bone. **Ligaments** are tough, fiber-like tissues that connect two or more bones, typically at a joint.

strain an injury that occurs when a muscle is stretched or "pulled" beyond its capacity.

sprain an injury that occurs when two or more bones that make up a joint are stretched beyond their capacity.

dislocation an injury that occurs when one or more bones that make up a joint become displaced.

10.4 Differentiate between an open and closed skeletal injury.

open fracture an injury in which the soft tissue of the skin has been broken at or near the fracture site.

closed fracture an injury in which the skin remains intact at the fracture site.

INJURIES TO THE MUSCULOSKELETAL SYSTEM

The different types of musculoskeletal injury that can occur are strain, sprain, fracture, and dislocation.

- **Strain.** A **strain** is an injury that occurs when a muscle is stretched or "pulled" beyond its capacity. Strains are relatively minor events and will usually heal on their own without advanced medical care.

- **Sprain.** A **sprain** injury occurs when two or more bones that make up a joint are stretched beyond their capacity. Sprains can cause damage to much of the soft tissue that surrounds the affected joint, including tendons and ligaments.

- **Fracture.** A fracture occurs when a bone becomes broken or cracked. It can range from a very minor crack in a bone to severe damage that shatters the bone into many pieces. The severity of a fracture is often determined by the mechanism of injury. The greater the force involved, the greater the damage will be.

- **Dislocation.** A **dislocation** injury occurs when one or more of the bones that make up a joint, such as a knee or elbow, become displaced.

 SAFETY CHECK

Musculoskeletal injuries often can include open wounds that are bleeding. As when assisting all injured persons, it is important to wear the proper personal protective equipment when providing care. ●

Fractures and dislocations can be further classified as either open or closed injuries (▼ Figure 10.2). An **open fracture** is one in which the soft tissue of the skin has been broken at or near the fracture site. A **closed fracture** is one in which the skin remains intact at the fracture site. You will never be expected to determine if the injury is an actual fracture or something less. Let the doctors make that determination.

It is important to always control the bleeding of an open injury before attempting to immobilize it. Use clean, sterile dressings to minimize contamination of the wound.

Figure 10.2 Musculoskeletal injuries may be open or closed.

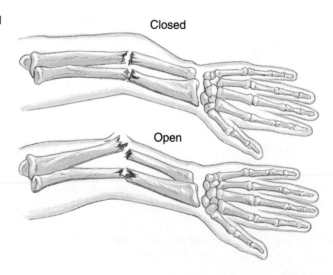

Closed

Open

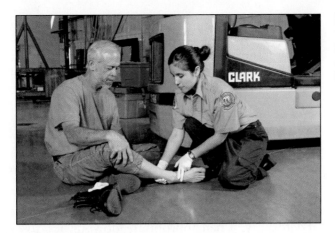

Figure 10.3 Determining the presence of a musculoskeletal injury is quite easy. If there is pain, there is an injury.

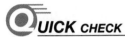UICK CHECK

Should bleeding from an open injury be controlled before or after the injured limb has been immobilized? ●

Signs and Symptoms of a Musculoskeletal Injury

Determining the presence of a musculoskeletal injury is quite easy. If there is pain, there is an injury. Determining the exact type of injury is another matter entirely (▲ Figure 10.3), but it is not your job to determine the exact nature of the injury, because that often requires the expertise of a physician with the assistance of x-rays and other diagnostic imaging equipment.

The first step in evaluating the injury is to understand the mechanism involved in causing it. In most situations, you must ask the person to describe what actually happened. Questions such as "How did the injury occur?" or "How did you land when you fell?" will help you determine the mechanism involved.

The signs and symptoms of a musculoskeletal injury include:

- Pain
- Deformity (swelling or angulation)
- Bruising
- Open wounds
- Exposed bone ends

The most common symptom of an injury is pain, but pain is not always a good indicator of how severe an injury might be. Some people have a high tolerance for pain and may not feel much even though the injury is significant. Ask the person if he can point with one finger to where it hurts the most. Do your best to determine if the pain is isolated to one location or if there is pain farther up or down from the injury site. You may have to use your gloved fingers to palpate (feel) the area below and above the injury site to determine where the pain begins and ends. Be very gentle and try not to cause unnecessary pain in the injured person.

10.5 Describe the signs and symptoms of a musculoskeletal injury.

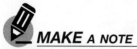

Even the fear of pain can cause a child to be very frightened and uncooperative. Be especially careful when performing an assessment of the injury, and tell the child everything you are doing. ●

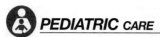 **MAKE** A NOTE

Because of the difficulty in knowing exactly what kind of injury a person may have, it is best to care for anyone with musculoskeletal pain as though the injury involves a broken bone. ●

angulation a deformity that occurs when a bone is broken and is bent out of its normal shape.

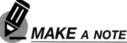 **QUICK** CHECK
What are two signs of deformity in a musculoskeletal injury? ●

10.6 Explain the priority of care for an injured person with a suspected open skeletal injury.

After determining the location of the pain, assess the injury site for signs of deformity. When appropriate, do your best to expose the injury by removing the clothing that covers it. If you need to cut clothing to expose the area, be sure to ask the person for permission first. If the injury involves the foot, it is helpful to loosen or remove the laces before attempting to remove the shoe. Observe for signs of deformity, which could include angulation and/or swelling (▼ Figure 10.4). **Angulation** occurs when a bone is broken and is bent out of its normal shape. Swelling occurs when the underlying soft tissues become damaged and bleeding occurs deep beneath the skin. Sometimes the bleeding is shallow and presents as a bruise, but bruises often can take hours to appear.

Next, you must assess the injury site for any evidence of an open wound. If you do find an open wound, you must control the bleeding using clean dressings and direct pressure. Be careful not to apply too much pressure, because this could cause more pain for the injured person. As you observe the wound, look for any evidence of broken bone ends. This will not change the care you provide, but it will be useful information for EMS personnel or other health-care providers when they arrive.

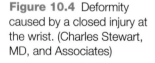 **MAKE** A NOTE

Your priority when caring for a musculoskeletal injury with an open wound is to control the bleeding before attempting to immobilize the injury site. ●

Figure 10.4 Deformity caused by a closed injury at the wrist. (Charles Stewart, MD, and Associates)

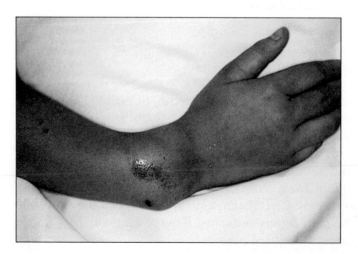

Assessing the Distal Extremity

One of the consequences of a skeletal injury to a leg or arm is damage to the blood vessels and nerves that run along the affected bone. For this reason it is important to assess the hand and foot properly when the injury involves a leg or arm bone.

Assess the hand and foot for the following characteristics:

- Circulation
- Sensation
- Movement

For all injuries to the extremities, you must do your best to determine if there is adequate circulation beyond the injury site by checking for the presence of **capillary refill**. You can check for capillary refill by squeezing the soft tissue of the big toe for a foot injury or by squeezing any finger in the case of an arm injury (▼ Figure 10.5). Squeezing the soft tissue causes the blood in the capillaries to be pushed out, making the skin appear blanched (whitish). Squeeze for a second or two, and then quickly release. You should see the

10.7 Explain the importance of an appropriate assessment of the distal extremity.

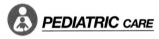 **PEDIATRIC** *CARE*

A child may be too frightened to move the hand or foot due to the fear of pain. ●

capillary refill the return of blood into capillaries after it has been forced out by fingertip pressure; normal refill time is two seconds.

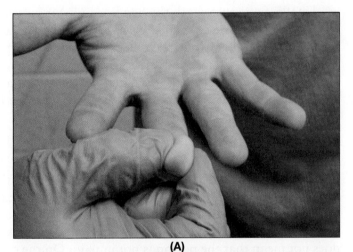

(A)

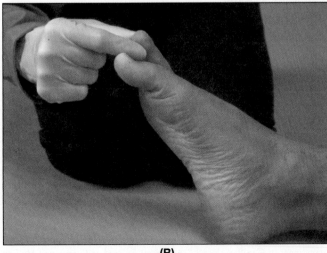

(B)

Figure 10.5 Check for distal circulation in the injured extremity by squeezing the soft tissue of the finger or toe until it blanches (pales). It should take no more than two seconds for the color to return to normal.

capillaries refill with blood and the tissue become pink again within two seconds. (This can be difficult to assess if lighting is poor.)[1]

If you should discover that capillary refill is slow or absent, take note of it. This will not change the care that you provide, but it is important information that should be passed on to EMS or other health-care providers because it will require advanced assessment and treatment. Be sure that anyone with compromised circulation seeks medical attention.

After circulation has been verified, check for normal sensation. With your gloved fingers, touch the fingers or toes of the injured extremity and ask if the person can feel your touch. You also will want to ask the person if the fingers or toes feel normal or if they feel numb or tingly.

Finally, you must check the hand or foot for movement. You can do this by asking the person to wiggle his toes or fingers. Ask if there is pain when he does this. If so, try to determine exactly where the pain is.

You will not change your care because of what you find during the assessment of circulation, sensation, and movement of an extremity. Your job is to document your findings and share them with the EMS or other health-care providers when they arrive to take over care.

Caring for Musculoskeletal Injuries

Due to the amount of pain that can be associated with musculoskeletal injuries, caring for someone with this type of injury can be challenging. In most instances, the injured person will have assumed a position that is most comfortable for his injury within a few seconds following the incident. This does not mean that the person is not in pain. On the contrary, he most likely is in a lot of pain.

The injured person will likely do whatever he can to keep the injured site from moving. This is often called "self-splinting." For instance, a person with an injured wrist or elbow will likely be holding the arm tightly against his body in an attempt to keep it from moving. This is the person's attempt to manually "splint" the injury.

In most instances you will be able to complete an adequate assessment of the injury while the person self-splints. This is preferred, because you do not want to cause any unnecessary movement.

If you have activated your Emergency Action Plan, called 911, the scene is safe, and no other injuries require emergency care, then there is no harm in simply allowing the injured person to self-splint and wait for EMS personnel

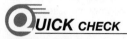
10.8 Explain the appropriate care for an injured person with a skeletal injury.

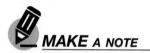
---

[1]L. H. Brown, N. H. Prasad, and T. W. Whitley, "Adverse Lighting Condition Effects on the Assessment of Capillary Refill," *American Journal of Emergency Medicine* 12 (January 1994): 46–7.

or other health-care providers to arrive. When possible, apply cold (a plastic bag or damp cloth filled with ice) to the injured area to decrease bleeding, swelling, and pain. To prevent cold injury, place a thin towel or cloth between the cold source and the skin and limit application to 20 minutes or less.

If EMS is delayed, provide **manual stabilization** by gently placing your hands above and below the injury site to limit movement and prevent further injury.[2] If EMS is not readily available, such as in a natural disaster, and you must move the injured person yourself, first apply some type of splint to the injury.

manual stabilization restriction of movement by the use of the injured person's or responder's own hands; also called self-splinting.

PEDIATRIC CARE

In many cases, it is best to allow the child to self-splint rather than risk causing more pain. Encourage the child to hold very still, and add a pillow or blanket for support if appropriate. ●

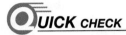
QUICK CHECK

When is "self-splinting" an acceptable method of stabilizing or immobilizing an injured extremity? ●

IMMOBILIZING A MUSCULOSKELETAL INJURY

A **splint** may be purchased commercially, or it may be improvised from such things as blankets, pillows, cardboard, and wood. Steps for immobilizing a musculoskeletal injury are as follows:

splint a device used to immobilize an injured extremity.

1. Expose and assess the injury site and surrounding area.
2. Assess circulation, sensation, and movement of the hand or foot.
3. Immobilize the injury site by using a splint.
4. Immobilize the joint above and below the injury site.
5. Reassess circulation, sensation, and movement.

Whenever possible, it will be important for the comfort of the injured person to keep the hand and/or foot in as natural a position as possible when immobilizing it to a splint. This is referred to as maintaining a **position of function**.

It should be noted that it is important to keep comfort in mind throughout the entire immobilization process. This means using adequate amounts of padding and minimizing excess movement of the injury site.

position of function the natural relaxed position of a body part, specifically the hand or foot.

Immobilizing a Long Bone Injury

The following technique is ideal for any long bone of the body, such as the bones of the upper arm, forearm, thigh, and lower leg. If the injury is angulated, stabilize the injury in the position found and wait for EMS personnel to arrive. For immobilizing long bone injuries, follow these guidelines (Scan 10.1):

- Thoroughly pad all rigid splints as appropriate.
- Make sure the splint extends well beyond the injury site on both sides as appropriate.

---

[2]American Heart Association, "2005 American Heart Association Guidelines for Cardiopulmonary Resuscitation and Emergency Cardiovascular Care, Part 14: First Aid: Musculoskeletal Trauma: Sprains, Strains, Contusions, and Fractures," *Circulation* 112 (2003): IV-196-IV-20, http://circ.ahajournals.org/cgi/content/full/112/24_suppl/IV-196 (accessed January 12, 2010).

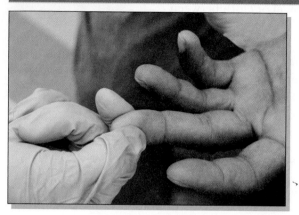

10.1.1 Assess circulation, sensation, and movement.

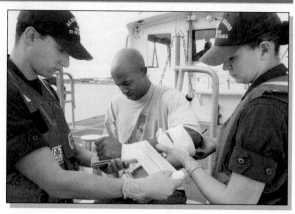

10.1.2 Extend the splint beyond the injury site on both sides. Secure it at each end. Add additional ties in the middle as needed.

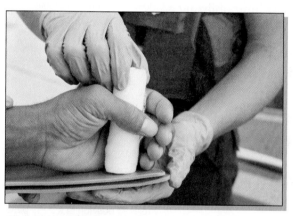

10.1.3 Keep the hand in the position of function. A roll of gauze or similar object in the person's hand will help.

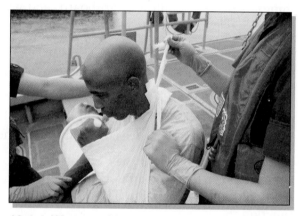

10.1.4 When possible, elevate the injury to help minimize pain. Add a sling to provide support.

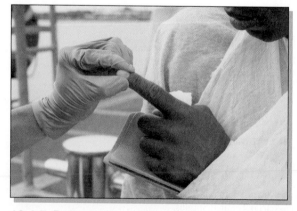

10.1.5 Reassess circulation, sensation, and movement.

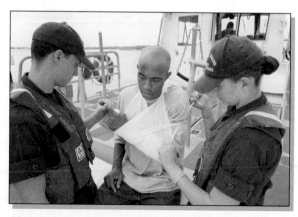

10.1.6 Add a swathe to help keep the limb secure against the body.

- Secure the rigid splint at each end first, and then add additional ties as needed in the middle.
- Keep the hand or foot in the position of function.
- When possible, elevate the injury to minimize pain.

Immobilizing a Joint Injury

Joint injuries have a greater potential for long-term disability because they occur where two or more bones come together. Joints also are the location for many blood vessels, nerves, tendons, and ligaments. The following technique is ideal for any joint, including the wrist, elbow, shoulder, or knee.

Follow these guidelines when immobilizing a *joint* injury (Scan 10.2 on page 146):

- Do not attempt to straighten the injury, because this could cause more damage.
- Immobilize the injury in the position found.
- Thoroughly pad all rigid splints as appropriate.
- Make sure the splint extends well beyond the injury site on both sides as appropriate.
- Secure rigid splints at each end first, and then add additional ties as needed in the middle.
- Keep the hand or foot in the position of function.
- When possible, elevate the injury to minimize pain.

You can use many things to secure a splint to an injured extremity. Roller gauze, tape, and cravats are some of the most common and convenient tools for this purpose. **Cravats** are simply triangular bandages that have been folded into a long, narrow strip, much like a bandana. Cravats have some advantages over other choices because they can be applied quickly and offer the most stability.

Application of a Sling and Swathe

A **sling** is a triangular cloth device used to immobilize an injured arm. It is ideal for nearly all arm injuries when the arm can be placed in the flexed position. A sling provides support for the arm, and, when used in conjunction with a **swathe**, it will allow for full immobilization of the arm and shoulder (▶ Figure 10.6). A swathe is a wide strip of cloth, typically formed from a folded triangular bandage that is used to secure an injured arm to the body. The swathe is applied after the sling and should be placed as low across the arm as possible. When properly placed, the swathe minimizes movement of the affected shoulder.

Follow these steps for application (Scan 10.3 on page 147):

1. Hold the sling by one end with the top of the triangle pointed toward the injured arm.
2. Slip the sling under the injured arm and place the top end of the sling over the uninjured (opposite) shoulder.

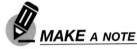

MAKE A NOTE

Do not attempt to straighten an injury to a joint. This could cause more pain and more damage to the structures that make up the joint. For most joint injuries, you will immobilize the injury in the position in which it is found. ●

cravat a triangular bandage that is folded to a width of about three inches and used to tie a splint or dressing in place.

sling a triangular cloth device used to immobilize an injured arm.

swathe a large cravat usually made of cloth, used to secure a sling or splint to the body.

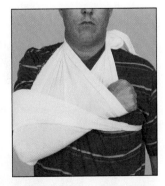

Figure 10.6 A sling and a swathe are ideal for nearly all arm injuries when the arm can be placed in the flexed position.

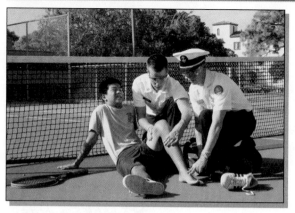

10.2.1 Assess distal circulation.

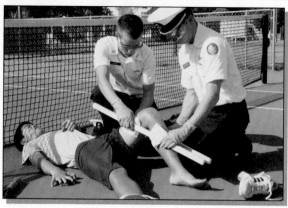

10.2.2 Apply a rigid splint to both sides of the leg near the knee.

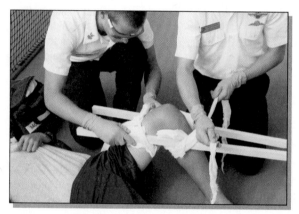

10.2.3 Secure the splint at both ends.

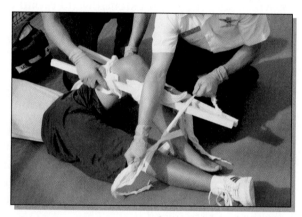

10.2.4 Secure the ankle of the injured leg to the uninjured leg.

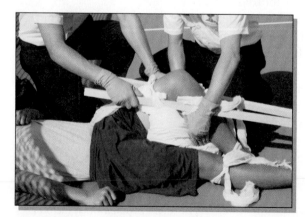

10.2.5 Place a towel or pillow under the injured knee for support.

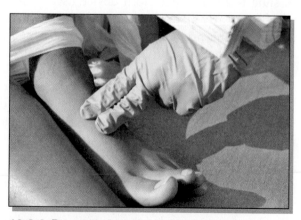

10.2.6 Reassess distal circulation, sensation, and motor function.

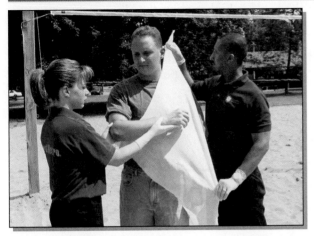

10.3.1 Hold the sling by one end with the top of the triangle pointed toward the injured arm. Slip the sling under the injured arm and place the top end of the sling over the uninjured (opposite) shoulder.

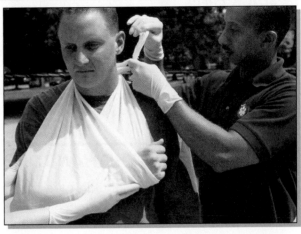

10.3.2 Bring the lower end of the sling up and over the injured arm and over the injured shoulder. Tie both long ends together at the side of the neck.

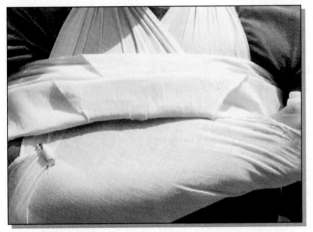

10.3.3 Adjust the sling so that the hand is higher than the elbow. Tie a knot, tape, or pin the opening at the elbow. Add a swathe to help keep the arm immobilized.

QUICK CHECK

In addition to self-splinting, manual stabilization, and splinting, what additional emergency care can be performed that will help decrease bleeding, swelling, pain, and disability? ●

3. Bring the lower end of the sling up and over the injured arm and over the injured shoulder.

4. Adjust the sling so that the hand is higher than the elbow.

5. Tie both long ends together at the side of the neck.

6. Tie a knot, tape, or pin the opening at the elbow.

7. Place a roll of gauze or similar object in the person's hand to maintain a position of function.

8. Pad the sling at the back of the neck for comfort.

THE HANDOFF

"Shouldn't we be splinting it or something?" Janet Grey, the school's principal, is standing above you and the girl, nervously clicking one high heel on the concrete.

"It's okay, Janet," you say, rubbing the student's shoulder. "It's an isolated injury and Jenny here is doing a great job holding it still. The ambulance should be here any minute."

"Do you think they're going to have to do surgery?" The girl looks at you, fear in her eyes as the sound of sirens starts to grow louder.

"I honestly don't know, Jenny, but I would doubt it. It looks like a pretty straightforward injury."

"My brother had to have surgery on his broken leg a few years ago, and he still has trouble walking sometimes."

"I really wouldn't worry about that." An ambulance, followed closely by a fire truck pulls into the school's circular driveway. "Let's just wait and see what the doctor says."

"What happened?" A uniformed EMT kneels next to you and the student.

"This is Jenny," you say. "She's fourteen with no medical history. She says that she slid down the stairs and when she got to the bottom she put her hand out to stop herself and now has a painful, swollen, and deformed left forearm. I decided to let her just hold it steady until you got here."

"Great decision," the EMT says to you before turning to Jenny. "Okay, Jenny, let's take a look at your arm.

CHAPTER REVIEW

Chapter Summary

- The musculoskeletal system is made up of two separate systems: the skeletal system, which comprises over 200 separate bones, and the muscular system, which is made up of the muscles and tendons.

- The musculoskeletal system has many functions, including support, movement, protection, and cell production.

- The four common types of musculoskeletal injuries are strains, which involve muscles; sprains, which occur at joints; fractures, which can occur with any bone; and dislocations, which also affect the joints.

- Musculoskeletal injuries can be classified as either open or closed injuries. With closed injuries, the skin above the injury site remains intact. With open injuries, the skin has become broken at or near the injury site.

- The signs and symptoms of a musculoskeletal injury include pain, deformity, bruising, open wounds, and exposed bone ends.

- The priority of care when managing a person with an open injury is to control all bleeding before attempting to immobilize the injury.

- Skeletal injuries can damage the vessels and nerves that run near the injury site. It is important to assess circulation (capillary refill), sensation, and movement of the hand or foot when appropriate.

- Self-splinting is an acceptable method for immobilizing an injury. If EMS personnel is delayed, perform manual stabilization by gently placing your hands above and below the injury site to limit movement and prevent further injury.

- If EMS personnel is not readily available and you must move the injured person yourself, splint the injury site as well as the joints above and below the injury site.

- When possible, apply cold to the injured area to decrease bleeding, swelling, and pain. Limit application to 20 minutes or less.

Quick Quiz

1. You respond to assist a woman who fell from a short stepladder. She is complaining of severe left knee pain and insists on keeping it bent at a 90-degree angle. One of your coworkers advises you to straighten the woman's leg prior to splinting. You should:

   a. immobilize her leg in the position found.

   b. straighten her leg before splinting.

   c. not immobilize her leg, since this could cause more pain.

   d. ask the person what she wants to do.

2. What does it mean when you pinch the soft tissue on the hand below an arm injury and the pinched skin stays blanched (pale)?

   a. That is normal for most serious arm injuries.

   b. There is a circulatory problem, and the person should seek advanced medical attention.

   c. The person should immediately be treated for shock.

   d. The person should be moved to a warmer environment.

3. When assessing the extremities distal to an injury site, you will be checking for_____, sensation, and movement.

   a. motor function

   b. turgidity

   c. pain

   d. circulation

4. All of the following are signs or symptoms of a musculoskeletal injury EXCEPT:

   a. deformity.

   b. bruising.

   c. sweating.

   d. pain.

5. When a muscle is stretched beyond its capacity it is called a:

   a. strain

   b. deformity

   c. sprain

   d. contusion

6. You arrive on the scene of a skateboard accident to find an upset boy lying on the ground. Blood is pouring steadily from an open injury of his right leg. After ensuring that his airway is open and his breathing is adequate, your next step is to:

   a. immobilize the joints above and below the open injury.

   b. stop the bleeding.

   c. perform a physical exam to assess for other injuries.

   d. question bystanders to determine exactly what occurred.

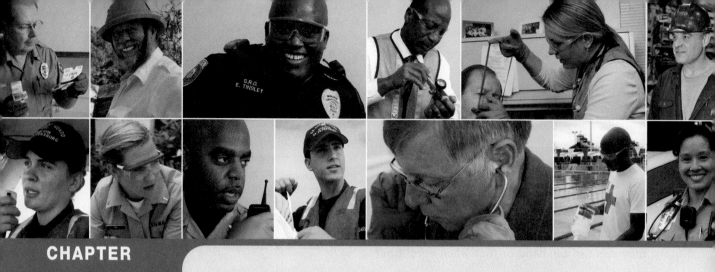

Caring for Injuries to the Head and Spine

KEY TERMS

The following terms are introduced in this chapter:

- central nervous system *(p. 152)*
- cervical spine *(p. 154)*
- coccyx *(p. 155)*
- cranium *(p. 151)*
- lumbar spine *(p. 155)*
- paralysis *(p. 155)*
- peripheral nervous system *(p. 155)*
- priapism *(p. 157)*
- sacrum *(p. 155)*
- thoracic spine *(p. 154)*

LEARNING OBJECTIVES

At the conclusion of this chapter and the associated instructor-guided lesson, the student will be able to:

Cognitive

11.1 Describe the major components of the cranium. *(p. 151)*

11.2 Differentiate between an open and closed head injury. *(p. 153)*

11.3 Describe the signs and symptoms of a head injury. *(p. 153)*

11.4 Explain the appropriate care for a person with a head injury. *(p. 154)*

11.5 Describe the major components of the spinal column. *(p. 154)*

11.6 Describe the major components of the nervous system. *(p. 155)*

11.7 Explain the relationship of the mechanism of injury to the potential for spinal injury. *(p. 155)*

11.8 Describe the signs and symptoms of a spinal injury. *(p. 157)*

11.9 Explain the appropriate care for a person with a suspected spinal injury. *(p. 157)*

11.10 Explain the special considerations of airway management for a person with suspected cervical spine injury. *(p. 154)*

Psychomotor

11.11 Demonstrate the care of a person with a head injury.)

11.12 Demonstrate the appropriate care for a person with a suspected spinal injury.

11.13 Demonstrate the proper airway management for a person with suspected spinal injury.

11.14 Demonstrate the proper technique for log-rolling an injured person.

11.15 Demonstrate the proper technique for manual stabilization of an injured person in a supine position.

11.16 Demonstrate the proper technique for manual stabilization of an injured person who is seated.

Introduction

INJURIES to the head and spine are very common and can lead to significant disability and death if not identified and managed appropriately. This chapter describes the common causes of head and spine injury as well as the proper techniques for assessment and care of someone who you suspect may have a head and/or spinal injury.

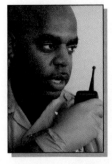

THE EMERGENCY

"Drivers," the announcer's voice booms over the loud speakers. "Start your engines!"

The string of amateur racers start their vehicles, filling the air with the thunderous din of high-powered machines and the pungent smell of gasoline. You have a great view of the track from where you are standing under the raised announcement platform, a dozen or so feet from your emergency-response pickup, which is packed with fire extinguishers, tools, and a medical kit.

The sparse crowd, mostly friends of the drivers, begins cheering as the light pole blinks down the line from red, through several yellows, and finally to green, which sends the eclectic collection of cars hurtling down the track in a cloud of blue-gray smoke. You watch the two lead cars battling for position into the first turn, bumping fenders and pulling away from the pack simultaneously on the back straightaway.

"And number 73 seems to be pulling away," the loudspeaker announces.

Just then, the number two car guns his engine and attempts to navigate the backside curve by cutting in close to the bottom of the track. You instinctively check your front pocket for the truck keys because you have seen this move before and it usually ends badly for one or more of the drivers.

As predicted, the car is going too fast on the turn and loses traction on the soft shoulder, sending a spray of dirt up onto the track. By the time the back end of the car swings up onto the track, sending the car sliding sideways, you are already halfway to the truck. As the car's tires suddenly grab the pavement, flipping the car over and over and sending pieces high into the air, you pop your truck into drive and speed across the grass toward the far side of the track.

As you arrive near the smoking devastation that used to be a car, you grab a fire extinguisher with one hand and the medical bag with the other. As you approach, you see the driver is pulling himself from the overturned vehicle, dragging his legs in a way that immediately makes you fear a spinal injury.

INJURIES TO THE HEAD

The **cranium,** or skull, comprises several bones that are fused together to form the cranial vault and face (▼ Figure 11.1). The cranial vault is the area inside the skull where the brain is located. The cranium sits at the top of the

11.1 Describe the major components of the cranium.

cranium the skull.

Figure 11.1 The bones of the human skull.

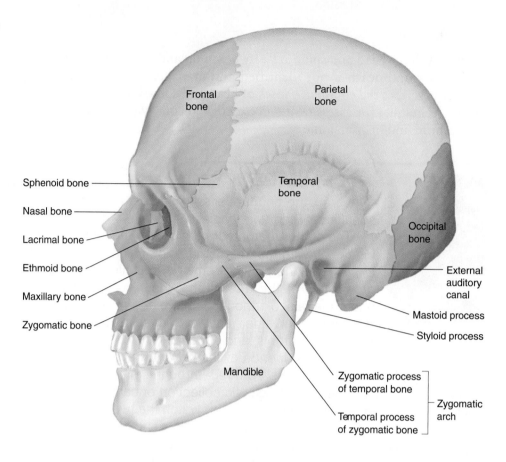

spinal column and is able to twist and move in many directions. It is this position and ability to move in all directions that makes the head and neck so susceptible to injury.

The brain and the spinal cord together make up the **central nervous system.** It is the central nervous system that is responsible for many of the body's involuntary functions, such as heartbeat, respirations, and temperature regulation. When the brain becomes injured, some or all of these important functions can be compromised.

Injuries to the head are commonly caused by blunt trauma. Blunt trauma can occur when an object strikes the head or when the head strikes a hard object, such as the ground after a fall or the inside of a vehicle during a traffic collision.

central nervous system the system that is responsible for involuntary functions, such as heartbeat, respirations, and temperature regulation; it is composed of the brain and the spinal cord.

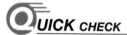

QUICK CHECK

Which part of the body is responsible for regulating many of the body's involuntary functions? ●

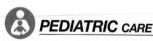

PEDIATRIC CARE

Young children are very prone to head injuries. One reason is that in children the head is proportionally large compared to the size of the body. This makes the head difficult to support and protect during falls. ●

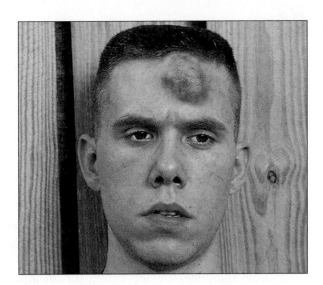

Figure 11.2 A closed head injury.

Head injuries can be either closed or open. Closed injuries occur when the cranium remains intact (▲ Figure 11.2). Open injuries occur when the cranium and overlying soft tissue are broken, exposing the brain and other soft tissues inside the skull. It is often difficult to determine if a head injury is open or closed because the soft tissues of the scalp can be damaged and bleeding without significant injury to the cranium. It is always best to assume that a head injury is open and to care for it accordingly.

Signs and Symptoms of Head Injury

Injuries to the head can range from minor lacerations to the scalp to severe skull fractures and significant injury to the brain. While it is difficult to know the true extent of damage when the head is injured, one of the best immediate indicators is the mental status of the injured person. A person who is alert and oriented following a head injury is likely to have less damage than a person who is unresponsive and bleeding.

The following is a list of common signs and symptoms of a head injury:

- Bleeding of the scalp
- Deformity of the cranium
- Altered mental status
- Unresponsiveness
- Nausea and vomiting
- Convulsions
- Abnormal vital signs
- Abnormal breathing patterns
- Combative behavior
- Repetitive questions

It is important to always consider the possibility of spinal injury when caring for a person with a head injury. The force sustained by the head also could have caused injury to the vertebrae of the neck.

11.2 Differentiate between an open and closed head injury.

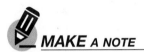

MAKE A NOTE

When controlling bleeding with direct pressure, be careful not to apply too much pressure against the skull. This could put pressure on the brain if the person has suffered a significant skull fracture. ●

11.3 Describe the signs and symptoms of a head injury.

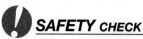
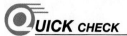

QUICK CHECK

A person with a head injury should be cared for as if he had what other type of injury? ●

Priorities of Care for Head Injuries

11.4 Explain the appropriate care for a person with a head injury.

11.10 Explain the special considerations of airway management for a person with suspected cervical spine injury.

When caring for someone with a head injury, it is important to suspect that he also may have suffered an injury to the vertebrae of the neck. Whenever possible, maintain manual stabilization of the head and neck when providing care.

Follow these steps when caring for an injured person with a suspected head injury:

1. Perform a primary assessment and ensure the ABCs (airway, breathing, circulation) are intact. If the person is unresponsive, open the airway with the jaw-thrust maneuver first. If this is unsuccessful, use the head-tilt/chin-lift method.

2. If necessary, provide rescue breaths using an appropriate barrier device.

3. Control any obvious bleeding. Be careful not to apply too much pressure to a head wound, because you may put pressure on the brain if the skull has been fractured.

4. Keep the person still and lying flat. Maintain manual stabilization of the head and neck.

5. Administer supplemental oxygen if available. Follow local protocols.

6. Have suction prepared in case the person vomits.

7. Monitor vital signs, including mental status.

MAKE A NOTE

Your first attempt at opening the airway of an unresponsive person with a head injury should be with the jaw-thrust maneuver. If the jaw-thrust does not open the airway, use the head-tilt/chin-lift maneuver. Maintaining an open airway and providing adequate ventilation is a critical priority. ●

QUICK CHECK

Why is the jaw-thrust maneuver preferred for an injured person with suspected neck injury? ●

INJURIES TO THE SPINE

11.5 Describe the major components of the spinal column.

cervical spine the neck bones; it is composed of seven vertebrae.

thoracic spine the middle segment of the spine; these bones articulate with the ribs; it is composed of 12 vertebrae.

The spinal column is made up of a series of stacked bones called vertebrae. Running down the center of the vertebrae is the spinal cord, which begins at the brain and runs down through the spinal column.

The spinal column is divided into the following major sections, beginning at the top (▶ Figure 11.3):

- **Cervical spine** (7 vertebrae)
- **Thoracic spine** (12 vertebrae)

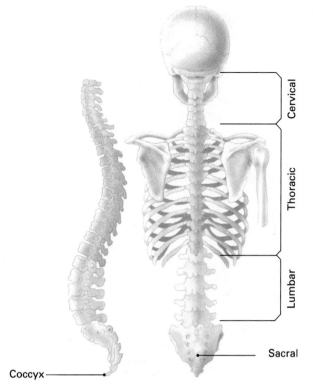

Figure 11.3 The spine.

Cervical

Thoracic

Lumbar

Sacral

Coccyx

- **Lumbar spine** (5 vertebrae)
- **Sacral spine** (5 vertebrae)
- **Coccyx**

The nervous system is divided into the central and the **peripheral nervous systems** (▼ Figure 11.4). The central nervous system is made up of the brain and spinal cord. The peripheral nervous system is made up of all the nerves and nerve endings that extend from the spinal cord throughout the body. When the spinal cord becomes damaged due to trauma, it can cause loss of sensation and **paralysis** to the areas of the body below the injury site. Cervical spinal cord injuries are rare but potentially catastrophic.

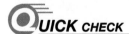
UICK CHECK

Which part of the spine is located in the neck and consists of seven vertebrae? ●

Mechanism of Injury

Sometimes the only evidence you may have of a possible spinal injury is the mechanism of injury (▼ Figure 11.5). It is especially important to evaluate and understand the exact mechanism involved so that you can provide the most appropriate care for the injured person.

Common mechanisms of injury that warrant a high suspicion for spinal injury occur when the person:

- Is involved in a motor vehicle, motorcycle/motor scooter, or bicycle crash as an occupant, rider, or pedestrian

lumbar spine the lower back and largest movable portion of the spine; it is composed of five vertebrae.

sacrum a triangular segment at the base of the spine; the upper part connects with the last lumbar vertebra and the bottom part with the coccyx; it is composed of five fused bones.

coccyx the tailbone, or final segment of the spinal column.

11.6 Describe the major components of the nervous system.

peripheral nervous system a body system that connects the CNS to the limbs and organs by way of nerves; it is composed of all the nerves and nerve endings that extend from the spinal cord throughout the body.

paralysis the loss of mobility.

11.7 Explain the relationship of the mechanism of injury to the potential for spinal injury.

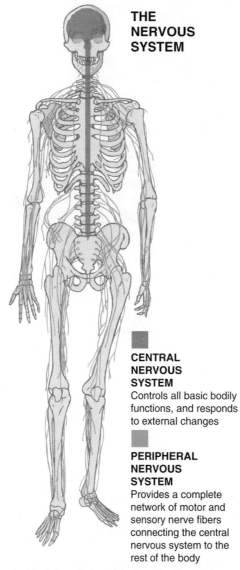

THE NERVOUS SYSTEM

CENTRAL NERVOUS SYSTEM
Controls all basic bodily functions, and responds to external changes

PERIPHERAL NERVOUS SYSTEM
Provides a complete network of motor and sensory nerve fibers connecting the central nervous system to the rest of the body

Figure 11.4 The central and peripheral nervous systems.

- Is injured as a result of a fall from greater than a standing height
- Complains of neck or back pain, tingling in the extremities, or weakness
- Is not fully alert
- Appears to be intoxicated
- Has a head or neck injury[1]

---

[1]American Heart Association, "2005 American Heart Association Guidelines for Cardiopulmonary Resuscitation and Emergency Cardiovascular Care, Part 14: First Aid: Injury Emergencies: Spine Stabilization," *Circulation* 112 (2005): IV-196–IV-203, http://circ.ahajournals.org/cgi/content/full/112/24_suppl/IV-196 (accessed January 12, 2010).

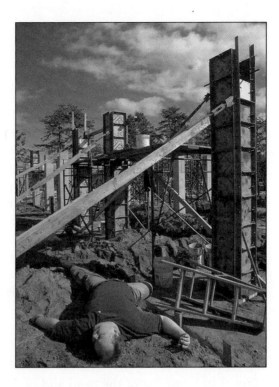

Figure 11.5 The mechanism of injury may be the only evidence you may have of a possible spinal injury.

Signs and Symptoms of Suspected Spinal Injury

The following is a list of the most common signs and symptoms of a spinal injury:

- Pain over the spine
- Deformity over the spine
- Numbness, weakness, or tingling in the extremities
- Loss of sensation
- Paralysis
- Incontinence (bladder or bowel)
- **Priapism** (erection of the penis)

Carefully check all extremities for circulation, sensation, and movement (CSM). Any problems with CSM can be an indication of a possible spinal injury. Not all spinal injuries are immediate or permanent. The spinal cord can be damaged by direct injury or by swelling that occurs hours after the injury. Damage also can occur during care and transport of the injured person. Be especially careful when assessing an injured person with suspected spinal injury.

Priorities of Care for Suspected Spinal Injury

Injuries to the spine can result in a wide range of severity. Do not be fooled by the absence of obvious signs and symptoms during your assessment. These injuries often will worsen as time passes, so be very diligent with your assessment.

When caring for an injured person with a suspected spinal injury, perform a primary assessment and ensure that the ABCs are intact. If you must

11.8 Describe the signs and symptoms of a spinal injury.

priapism persistent erection of the penis secondary to spine injury.

11.9 Explain the appropriate care for a person with a suspected spinal injury.

manage the airway, attempt the jaw-thrust maneuver first, before the head-tilt/chin-lift maneuver. Then manually stabilize the head so that the head, neck, and spine do not move and are kept in line.

If additional Emergency Responders are available, perform a patient assessment including all extremities. Obtain and monitor vital signs. Provide supplemental oxygen, if available, following local protocols.

You should be aware that not all injured people will present with obvious signs and symptoms of a spinal injury. Those with altered mental status and those who appear intoxicated are not able to reliably report pain. Sometimes signs and symptoms do not appear for hours. So any injured person who appears intoxicated, has an altered mental status, or is found unresponsive should be cared for as though he has a spinal injury.

 MAKE A NOTE

If you find an unresponsive person and are unable to determine an exact mechanism of injury or nature of illness, you should care for the person as though he has a spinal injury. ●

Manual Stabilization

Manual stabilization of the head and neck is an important step in caring for an injured person with a suspected spinal injury. There are two basic approaches to an injured person who is supine (lying face up). One is approaching the person from the side and placing your hand on his forehead to minimize movement. The second is kneeling at the top of the person's head and using both hands to grasp the head from the sides (Scan 11.1). If the person is injured and his head is turned to one side or the other, and he is alert and breathing well, it is best to manually stabilize the head in the position found. If you have any reason to suspect the person is not breathing adequately, you must carefully move the head so that it is aligned with the body and confirm he has a clear and open airway.

| **SCAN 11.1** | **Manual Stabilization of Head and Neck** |

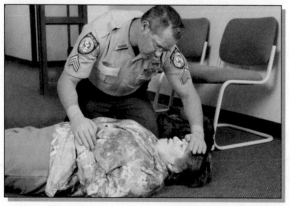

11.1.1 Using one hand to provide manual stabilization of the head when you are at the side of the injured person.

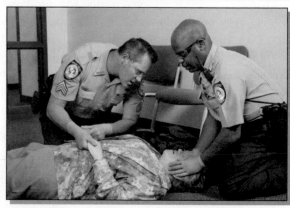

11.1.2 Using two hands to provide manual stabilization of the injured person's head and neck.

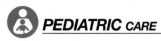
Children have a very large posterior skull. This can cause the head to tilt forward when they are placed in a supine position. Carefully slipping a folded towel under the shoulders will help keep the head and neck in a more neutral position. ●

To perform manual stabilization of the head and neck of a supine person, follow these steps:

1. Kneel at the top or side of the injured person's head.
2. Introduce yourself, and explain to the person what you are going to do.
3. Grasp the person's head by placing your hands firmly on each side of the head, and hold firmly.
4. Instruct the person to remain still and provide reassurance.
5. Monitor the ABCs by talking to the person and listening to how he responds.

Follow these steps for performing manual stabilization of the head and neck of a seated person (▼ Figure 11.6):

1. Stand or sit directly behind the injured person.
2. Introduce yourself, and explain to the person what you are going to do.
3. Grasp the person's head by placing your hands firmly on each side of the head, and hold firmly.
4. Instruct the person to remain still and provide reassurance.
5. Monitor the ABCs by talking to the person and listening to how he responds.

Performing a Log Roll

Occasionally, it may be necessary to roll an injured person from his back onto his side or from his stomach to his back. This may be required to help manage the airway or assist in moving him onto a long spine board for immobilization. While this can be performed with fewer than three rescuers, it is best performed with three.

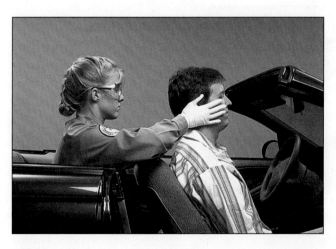

Figure 11.6 Manually stabilizing the head and neck of a seated person.

To roll an ill or injured person onto his side, follow these steps (Scan 11.2):

1. One responder should kneel at the top of the ill or injured person's head and hold or stabilize the head and neck in the position it is found.
2. A second responder should kneel at the person's side.
3. A third responder should kneel next to the person's legs.
4. Responders should grasp the person's shoulders, hips, and knees.
5. The responder at the person's head should signal and give directions. For example, "On the count of three, slowly roll. One, two, three—roll together."
6. In response, all responders should slowly roll the person in a coordinated move, carefully keeping the spine in a neutral, in-line position until the person is supine.

You may have to roll an ill or injured person onto his side to check for and control bleeding from the back or perhaps to help clear the airway if he

| SCAN 11.2 | **Performing a Log Roll** |

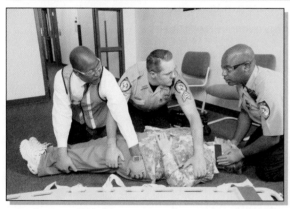

11.2.1 One responder should kneel at the top of the ill or injured person's head and hold or stabilize the head and neck in the position found.

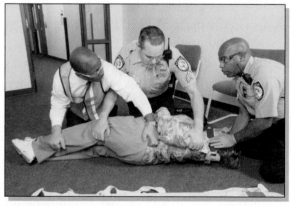

11.2.2 At a signal from the rescuer at the head, all responders should slowly roll the person toward them in a coordinated move.

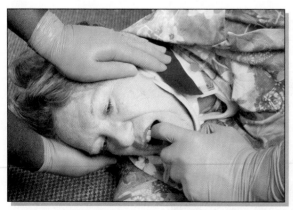

11.2.3 One reason to perform a log roll is to clear the injured person's airway.

vomits. To reverse the roll and return the person to the supine position, allow the person at the head to call the move and gently roll the person back down, being sure to keep the spine in alignment at all times.

THE HANDOFF

Just as you reach the injured driver, he slides to the ground, rolls over onto his back, and pulls his cracked helmet off.

"Hold on. Stop moving," you say, kneeling in the grass and holding his head in a neutral, in-line position.

"My back is killing me, and I can't feel my legs," he says between heavy, pained breaths. "What happened?"

"You wrecked your car." You look directly down into his eyes so he isn't tempted to turn his head. "You're injured and need to stay still. An ambulance is coming across the track right now."

"What happened?" He asks again, obviously unaware that you just answered that question.

"You were in a car crash, and I need you to stay completely still. Does anything hurt besides your back?"

"My head," the man says, reaching up and touching his dirty forehead. "Here."

Within moments an EMT and a Paramedic are at your side, unzipping bags and positioning a long spine board next to the driver.

"What do you have for me?" The Paramedic asks while checking the driver's radial pulse.

"Well," you say. "He was in that car over there that flipped several times coming out of the turn. He's complaining of back and head pain, was dragging his legs, and said he couldn't feel them."

"What happened to me?" the driver interrupts.

"And he's confused," you say before looking back down at the driver. "You were in a car crash."

"I'm really glad that you decided to hold c-spine," the paramedic says, sizing a cervical collar while the EMT places an oxygen mask on the driver's face. "Do you think that you can help us get him packaged on the board?"

"Absolutely," you say proudly. "Anything you need."

CHAPTER REVIEW

Chapter Summary

- Open head injuries are those that result in a break in the bone and the overlying soft tissue. A closed head injury involves no opening of the skull, but there may be soft tissue damage of the scalp.

- Head injuries can range from a very mild concussion to significant open fractures of the skull. A person with a head injury often will have signs and symptoms ranging from a mild headache to bleeding of the scalp, altered mental status, deformity of the cranium, unresponsiveness, convulsions, and vomiting. Someone with a head injury also may display aggressive behavior and ask repetitive questions.

- Your first concern when caring for a person with a suspected head injury is to manage and monitor the ABCs. Consider the possibility of a neck injury and provide care accordingly. Control bleeding as appropriate.

- Management of the airway in an unresponsive person with a suspected neck injury can be challenging, but it is important to remember that the airway is always the top priority. If you must open the airway of an unresponsive injured person with a suspected neck injury, begin with the jaw-thrust maneuver. If the jaw-thrust maneuver is unsuccessful, use the head-tilt/chin-lift maneuver.

- When caring for a person with a suspected spinal injury, you must first try to identify the mechanism of injury. Always assume there is a spinal injury if the mechanism suggests it, even if the injured person has no obvious signs or symptoms.

- A person with a spinal injury may have pain and/or deformity over the injury site. He also may present with numbness, tingling, weakness of the extremities, loss of sensation, paralysis, and incontinence.

- Once you have confirmed that the ABCs are intact, your primary concern becomes stabilization of the head, neck, and spine. Provide manual stabilization of the head and neck until EMS arrives and is able to place the patient onto a long spine board.

Quick Quiz

1. What is the most important initial step that you can take when caring for a person with a suspected spinal injury?
   a. Assess the patient for circulation, sensation, and movement.
   b. Determine the mechanism of injury.
   c. Transport the patient to the nearest trauma center.
   d. Manually stabilize the patient's head and neck.

2. Which one of the following mechanisms of injury would cause you to suspect spinal injury?
   a. Circular saw amputation of fingers
   b. Fall from an anchored speedboat
   c. Bicycle crash
   d. Self-inflicted gunshot wound to the hip

3. You are requested to assist with an unresponsive person who was found facedown on a hotel lobby floor. How would you choose to move the patient into the recovery position?
   a. Two-person extremity lift
   b. Three-person log roll
   c. With a stair chair
   d. It would be better to wait for EMS.

4. Your patient is unresponsive following a motorcycle crash on the interstate. You find that he is not breathing, and you try to open his airway with the jaw-thrust maneuver but are not successful. What should you do next?

   a. Maintain manual stabilization and wait for EMS to arrive.
   b. Attempt the head-tilt/chin-lift maneuver.
   c. Attempt to ventilate the patient anyway.
   d. Begin chest compressions.

5. Combative behavior, abnormal breathing patterns, and repetitive questions are all signs of a(n):
   a. cervical spine injury.
   b. unresponsive person.
   c. peripheral nervous system trauma.
   d. injury to the head.

6. You witness a low-speed ATV collision at a local recreational area that knocks both riders from their vehicles. Neither of the men is wearing a helmet, and both quickly get back to their feet. You notice one of them is walking oddly as he retrieves his vehicle. You ask if he is okay, and he tells you that his legs "just feel really heavy." You should suspect:
   a. head injury.
   b. internal bleeding.
   c. spine injury.
   d. hip dislocation.

7. What are the two main components of the central nervous system?
   a. Peripheral and central nerves
   b. Discs and vertebrae
   c. Brain and spinal cord
   d. Spine and nerves

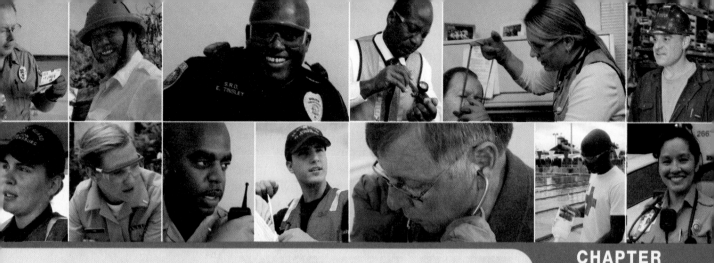

Multiple-Casualty Incidents and Principles of Triage

LEARNING OBJECTIVES

At the conclusion of this chapter and the associated instructor-guided lesson, the student will be able to:

Cognitive

12.1 Explain the criteria for a multiple-casualty incident. *(p. 165)*

12.2 Explain common causes of multiple-casualty incidents. *(p. 165)*

12.3 Explain the role of the Emergency Responder in the multiple-casualty situation. *(p. 165)*

12.4 Explain the goal and structure of an incident management system. *(p. 166)*

12.5 Explain the principles of triage at a multiple-casualty incident. *(p. 167)*

12.6 Differentiate the assessment criteria of the START triage system. *(p. 168)*

Psychomotor

12.7 Demonstrate the ability to properly categorize the ill or injured in a simulated multiple-casualty situation.

KEY TERMS

The following terms are introduced in this chapter:

- incident command system (ICS) *(p. 166)*
- multiple-casualty incident (MCI) *(p. 165)*
- national incident management system (NIMS) *(p. 166)*
- START triage system *(p. 168)*

Introduction

IT can be frightening enough to think about caring for a single person who is experiencing a sudden illness or injury, but the thought of having to care for several people at once can be overwhelming. While it does not happen very often, incidents that involve two, three, or more people can happen at any time, and it is important to know how they should be managed. This chapter introduces you to the basic concepts of managing a multiple-casualty incident and the principles involved with triage.

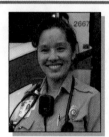

THE EMERGENCY

The bus is full but strangely quiet as it rolls along the highway toward the state prison complex in Bullrush County. You are part of the transportation team that picks up prison-bound inmates from various county detention centers around the western part of the state and delivers them to the appropriate facilities. The interior of the bus is divided into four caged sections: one for the driver; one large, seated section for the inmates; and guard boxes at the front and rear.

You are seated on a worn metal bench at the back of the bus, keys jangling at every bump in the road. You look out the window at the passing prairie lands as often as you look at the inmates sitting silently side by side in front of you.

Suddenly you see the driver spinning the large wheel, causing the bus to veer violently to the right. The guard in the front box braces for some kind of impact. Before you can even wonder what is happening, the front grill and windshield of a semi truck appears right in front of the bus and everyone is thrown heavily forward as the impact smashes the two vehicles together. You see the demolished cab of the semi, smoke pouring from the engine, compacting the front of the bus and pushing twisting metal infused with bodies back toward you. The sound of the collision and the inmates yelling is suddenly deafening, and you are vaguely aware that a fire has started somewhere toward the front of the tangled mess.

You kick the side door open and quickly climb down to the asphalt highway, stumbling back away from the huge, smoking wreck that has combined a full-sized bus and a big rig with a 53-foot trailer into one bulging mass. Inmates are screaming at you from the windows, some are breaking the glass and pushing at the bars lining the frames, and some appear dazed, blood running freely down their faces. You look up and down the highway and see no other vehicles between you and the horizon in either direction, making you suddenly feel very alone.

You pull your cell phone from your duty belt and force your hands to stop shaking so you can dial 911.

MULTIPLE-CASUALTY INCIDENTS

At first glance, the definition of the term **multiple-casualty incident** (MCI) seems obvious. It is an incident with more than one ill or injured person. While this is indeed true, the full definition involves more than simply the number of victims involved.

A more thorough definition of an MCI is any incident that overwhelms the normal Emergency Responders or resources. Most teams, agencies, or departments are more than prepared for a single person, and most prepare for two, three, and even four victims. Given the fact that a typical EMS response involves no fewer than three firefighters and two ambulance crewmembers, they are usually prepared for all but the most extreme events.

An incident at a factory or office building that involves two or more ill or injured people can easily overwhelm Emergency Responder resources and thus will require a slightly different approach to managing everyone at the scene. When you discover that you are responding to an incident that involves multiple ill or injured people, you must do your best to estimate the number involved and to request additional resources through the 911 system.

Scene Safety

By their very nature, incidents that affect multiple people are likely to be hazardous to those responding to the scene. Common causes of MCIs include:

- Explosion
- Wildfire
- Building collapse
- Earthquake
- Flood
- Hurricane
- Hazardous chemical spill
- Terrorist attack
- Mass shooting
- Vehicle collision

You must be especially careful when approaching the scene of an MCI. You will want to understand as best you can the mechanism involved *before* you get near or enter the scene.

 SAFETY CHECK

As with any scene, your personal safety is your primary concern. You are never obligated to put yourself at undue risk to perform emergency care. Sometimes your job is to remain clear of the scene and help ensure that others do not enter and become injured. ●

The Role of the Emergency Responder

As strange as it may seem, your role at the scene of an MCI may not involve caring for ill or injured people, at least not at first (▼ Figure 12.1). There may

---

12.1 Explain the criteria for a multiple-casualty incident.

multiple-casualty incident (MCI) an incident with more than one ill or injured person; any incident that overwhelms the normal Emergency Responders or resources.

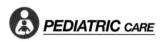 **PEDIATRIC** CARE

Incidents involving even a few children can easily overwhelm the local resources necessary to properly care for them. Many rural hospitals do not have the expertise to adequately care for significant illnesses and injuries involving children. ●

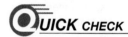 **UICK** CHECK

What is the commonly accepted definition of the term *multiple-casualty incident?* ●

12.2 Explain common causes of multiple-casualty incidents.

12.3 Explain the role of the Emergency Responder in the multiple-casualty situation.

Figure 12.1 MCI involving a school bus.

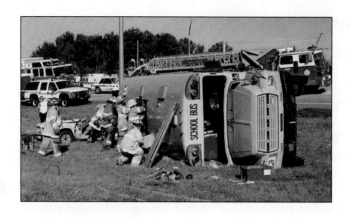

be more important duties, which are to evaluate the scene and identify and mitigate safety hazards before you ever approach an ill or injured person. Once you have confirmed that there are multiple victims involved, you must notify the 911 dispatcher. Provide as much information about the incident as you can. This will allow the dispatcher to send the appropriate resources to manage the scene and all of the ill or injured.

Next, for your own safety, you may have to remain clear of the scene as well as keep others from entering it. If there are hazards at the scene that have not been addressed, anyone who enters could become a victim.

If you are familiar with the area or building and its contents, you may be very helpful as a resource for EMS providers when they arrive. Once the scene has been rendered safe, then and only then, will you be expected to assist with the care and management of those who have been affected by the incident.

Overview of the Incident Command System (ICS)

The concept of an **incident command system (ICS)**, sometimes referred to as an incident management system (IMS), first originated back in the early 1970s following a series of devastating wildfires in southern California. Since that time, the system has grown to be a sophisticated structure that includes elements of command, operations, planning, logistics, and finance. The goal of ICS is to meet the needs of the incident in a fast and efficient manner by using an organized approach to command as well as to the appropriate use of resources.

In response to the increase in terrorist threats across the nation, the federal government has developed a nationwide system called the **national incident management system (NIMS)**. NIMS is a nationally standardized system developed by the federal government for managing large-scale incidents that involve multiple agencies. Emergency Responders and EMS personnel are required to train on how it functions.

For now, all you need to know is that once the fire department arrives at the scene of an MCI, fire personnel will take control of the incident by designating an Incident Commander, who will coordinate all of the resources needed to appropriately respond to the incident. As someone who has emergency medical training, you may become one of the resources utilized by the Incident Commander to triage and care for the ill or injured at the scene.

QUICK CHECK

What responsibilities do you have as an Emergency Responder at the scene of an MCI? ●

12.4 Explain the goal and structure of an incident management system.

incident command system (ICS) an organized approach to dealing with a multiple-casualty incident.

national incident management system (NIMS) a nationally standardized system developed by the federal government for managing large-scale incidents that involve multiple agencies.

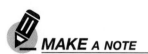

MAKE A NOTE

The federal government has developed a standardized system for managing large-scale incidents. It is called the national incident management system (NIMS). All Emergency Responders, EMS, and fire personnel are required to receive training on how this system works in the event of an incident. ●

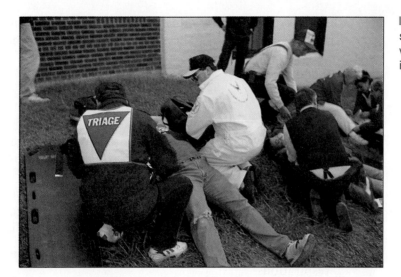

TRIAGE

In a perfect world, emergency services would be able to immediately dispatch enough responders to care for each and every ill or injured person at an MCI, one on one. This, of course, is not possible or efficient. To appropriately manage multiple ill or injured individuals at any scene, a process must be utilized so that the available resources can care for as many victims as possible. This process is called triage (▲ Figure 12.2). The word *triage* comes from the French word *trier*, which means "to sort."

12.5 Explain the principles of triage at a multiple-casualty incident.

Components of a Triage System

At the scene of an MCI, when there are more victims than medical personnel to provide care, responders must sort the ill and injured into groups according to condition. The idea is that only the people with the most critical injuries who have the best chance of survival will receive immediate care. In a typical triage system, the ill and injured will be quickly evaluated and categorized as one of the following:

- **Minor.** These people are often the "walking wounded" at the scene.
- **Delayed.** These are people who are not in immediate threat of dying and can wait for medical care.
- **Immediate.** These are people who must receive immediate attention or risk dying.
- **Deceased.** These are people who have no signs of life and would require multiple resources to attempt resuscitation. Doing so would put many others at risk.

Triaging ill or injured people is no easy task, especially when you have been trained to provide care to anyone who needs it. During the triage process, your goal is to quickly evaluate each and every person without providing any specific care. Only after you have identified and categorized all of the ill and injured will you begin to provide specific care.

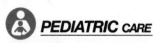
PEDIATRIC CARE

When dealing with MCIs involving children, do whatever you can to keep the children together with their parents or caregivers. This will help minimize the anxiety that such an event can cause for a young child. ●

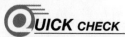

QUICK *CHECK*
According to a basic triage system, which of the ill or injured would be categorized as deceased? ●

12.6 Differentiate the assessment criteria of the START triage system.

START triage system a structured approach to triaging multiple injured individuals based on specific criteria.

During the triage process, others may be setting up treatment areas for each of the triage categories. The ill and injured will be moved to one of those areas based on their triage category and receive care specific to each one's chief complaint.

START Triage System

The **START triage system** is one of the more common triage systems in use today and has been proven useful in prioritizing transport of the most critically ill or injured people to area hospitals.[1]

The acronym START stands for Simple Triage And Rapid Treatment. The START triage system is a structured approach to categorizing multiple ill or injured individuals based on three specific criteria (▼ Figure 12.3):

R – *Respirations.* Each person is evaluated for the presence and rate of respirations.

Figure 12.3 The START triage decision tree.

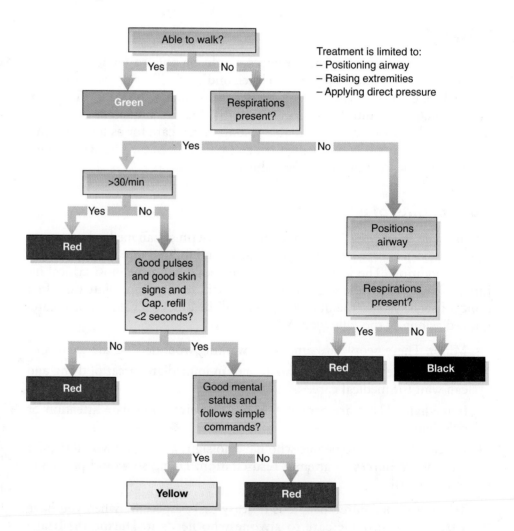

[1]C. A. Kahn, C. H. Schultz, K. T. Miller, and C. L. Anderson, "Does START Triage Work? An Outcomes Assessment after a Disaster," *Annals of Emergency Medicine* 54 (September 2009):424–30, 430.e1. Epub 2009 Feb 5.

P – *Perfusion status.* If respirations are adequate, perfusion status is evaluated using the capillary refill test. (Perfusion is the adequate supply of blood and oxygen to the tissues of the body.)

M – *Mental status.* Each person is evaluated for his or her ability to follow simple verbal commands.

There are a couple of important concepts that will help you when faced with a triage situation. First, you must "start where you stand." Begin triaging those ill and injured individuals closest to you and work your way through the scene from there. Do not move around looking for the worst person to begin with. The second important concept is to verbally direct all those who are able to walk to move to a safe area and sit down. This will allow some people to self-triage as "walking wounded," and it will help to clear the scene.

You always can use some of the walking wounded to assist you with providing care or accessing some of the more critically wounded. If you are triaging correctly, you will spend between 30 and 60 seconds with each person before tagging each one and moving on to the next person. Triage tags (▼ Figure 12.4) are tied to each person with the appropriate category showing at the bottom of the tag. Tags are designed so that the category can be changed should the person's condition worsen.

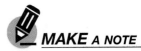

MAKE A NOTE

A quick tip that will help speed up the triage process is that all unresponsive people who are breathing can be immediately categorized as "Immediate." ●

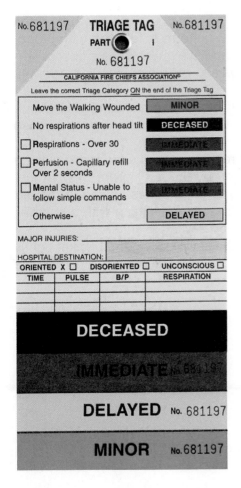

Figure 12.4 Example of a typical triage tag, front and back.

There is a variety of formal triage systems in use around the country. The START system is only one example of a structured method for sorting many ill or injured individuals. It will be important for you to learn the system that is in use in your area and understand what your role will be in the event of an MCI.

THE HANDOFF

"Everyone who can walk needs to get out now!" You yell above the pandemonium as you unlock the cage door at the back of the bus. "Climb down and get off of the highway."

You are momentarily pushed aside by a rush of yelling, bleeding, and limping men in bright orange jumpsuits shoving to get off of the smoky bus. As you stand at the back of the now mostly empty bus, you see that both drivers, the front guard, and several inmates are obviously deceased. There are still six inmates lying unmoving in the main cage who did not respond to your instructions to leave and whose injuries are not obvious. You hesitate for a moment and then step forward into the inmate area to begin triaging the six men.

Within about 20 minutes of your 911 call, the collision scene is growing busy with emergency vehicles, and you hear the rhythmic thumping of approaching helicopters.

"I am so glad to see you guys," you say as you climb down from the back of the bus, your exam gloves and uniform splattered with blood. "There are seven deceased at the front and five guys who are critically injured in the midsection. I opened airways and got major bleeding stopped, but that's all I could do."

"That's okay." A highway patrolman puts his arm around your shoulders. "We'll take care of them. We've got a convoy of ambulances and two choppers inbound."

As you sit on the polished chrome rear bumper of a fire truck, gulping breaths of oxygen, you are suddenly hit by the full impact of what just happened. A firefighter who is tending to the inmates seated in the dirt along the side of the highway notices that you are sitting with both arms across your chest, shaking, and comes over with a blanket.

"You did amazing work out here," she says, pulling the blanket tightly around you. "You kept your head in a horrible situation, and some of these guys owe you their lives."

CHAPTER REVIEW

Chapter Summary

- A multiple-casualty incident (MCI) is any event where the number of ill or injured overwhelms the Emergency Responders or resources.

- Explosions, wildfires, building collapses, earthquakes, floods, hurricanes, terrorist attacks, mass shootings, hazardous materials spills, and vehicle collisions are all common causes of MCIs.

- As an Emergency Responder at the scene of an MCI you may need to address issues of scene safety before you can begin caring for victims. Do your best to identify the cause of the incident while remaining at a safe distance. Activate your Emergency Action Plan or call 911 immediately with all available information.

- An incident command system (ICS) is a formalized structure that addresses the elements of command, operations, planning, logistics, and finance. The goal of ICS is to bring an organized approach to dealing with the incident in a fast and efficient manner.

- Triage is the process of "sorting" all ill and injured people at an MCI based on their immediate need for care and their likelihood for survival. The START triage system involves categorizing each person based on the criteria of respirations, perfusion, and mental status.

Quick Quiz

1. Most triage systems use all of the following categories EXCEPT:
   a. stable.
   b. deceased.
   c. minor.
   d. immediate.

2. The individual responsible for directing all resources during an MCI is called the:
   a. Battalion Chief.
   b. Incident Coordinator.
   c. MCI Director.
   d. Incident Commander.

3. You are the first to arrive at the scene of a passenger train derailment and see injured people scattered along both sides of the tracks. Once you have called 911 and requested an appropriate EMS response, which individuals should you start triaging first?
   a. The most critically ill or injured person
   b. The ones who have a pulse but no respirations
   c. The ones closest to where you stand
   d. The ones with severe bleeding

4. A multiple-casualty incident is not defined by the number of ill or injured individuals but by whether it:
   a. meets the definition detailed in the FEMA 300 course.
   b. overwhelms the initial responding resources.
   c. involves more than three people or vehicles.
   d. requires the use of a triage sorting system.

5. You pull into the parking lot of the chemical plant where you work as a safety officer and see several people lying on the ground near the entrance. You should do all of the following EXCEPT:
   a. immediately call 911.
   b. try to safely determine the cause of the problem.
   c. stay a safe distance from the incident area.
   d. assess the unresponsive people on the ground.

6. The letters in the popular triage system START stand for:
   a. Simple Triage And Rapid Treatment
   b. Start Triage And Request Transportation
   c. Simple Triage And Rapid Transport
   d. Start Treatment And Rapid Triage

7. When utilizing the START system, you would evaluate an individual's mental status by asking him:
   a. questions about current events.
   b. to follow simple verbal commands.
   c. to determine the next number in a sequence.
   d. questions for personal information, such as birthday.

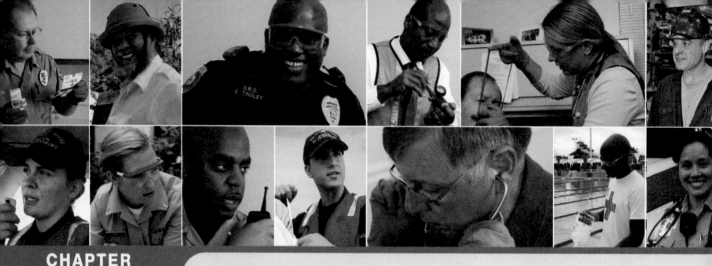

Childbirth

KEY TERMS

The following terms are introduced in this chapter:

- amniotic fluid *(p. 174)*
- amniotic sac *(p. 174)*
- birth canal *(p. 176)*
- breech birth *(p. 181)*
- cervix *(p. 175)*
- contractions *(p. 175)*
- crowning *(p. 176)*
- fallopian tube *(p. 174)*
- fetus *(p. 174)*
- imminent birth *(p. 175)*
- labor *(p. 175)*
- ovary *(p. 174)*
- placenta *(p. 174)*
- placenta previa *(p. 181)*
- prolapsed cord *(p. 181)*
- trimester *(p. 174)*
- umbilical cord *(p. 174)*
- uterus *(p. 174)*

LEARNING OBJECTIVES

At the conclusion of this chapter and the associated instructor-guided lesson, the student will be able to:

Cognitive

13.1 Describe the anatomy of pregnancy. *(p. 174)*

13.2 Describe the three stages of labor and when each begins and ends. *(p. 174)*

13.3 Describe the signs and symptoms of an imminent delivery. *(p. 175)*

13.4 Explain the steps for assisting with a field delivery. *(p. 177)*

13.5 Explain the priorities of care for the infant following a field delivery. *(p. 180)*

13.6 Explain the priorities of care for the mother following a field delivery. *(p. 181)*

13.7 Explain the common complications related to a field delivery and how to properly care for each. *(p. 181)*

Psychomotor

13.8 Demonstrate the steps for preparing for and assisting with a field delivery.

13.9 Demonstrate the proper care of the infant following a field delivery.

13.10 Demonstrate the proper care of the mother following a field delivery.

13.11 Demonstrate the ability to identify a complicated delivery.

13.12 Demonstrate the proper assessment and care for a complicated field delivery.

Introduction

WITNESSING the birth of a human being is one of the most amazing miracles of life and one that many people get to experience sometime during their lifetime. The vast majority of these events are anticipated and planned for and occur with few or no complications. However, there are some births that occur sooner than expected and often in a location that is not part of the overall plan. When these situations occur, it is often up to the Emergency Responder to assess the situation, attempt to gain control, and bring organization to an otherwise chaotic scene.

It is important to understand that just because a birth may occur outside of a hospital it does not mean it is a true medical emergency. Certainly the family may think so, and you should respond accordingly through your actions and words. In the absence of any known complications, the likelihood of a normal birth is quite good. This chapter introduces you to the process for assessing a woman in labor and the steps for assisting a normal birth.

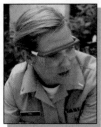

THE EMERGENCY

"Flight attendants, please secure doors," the pilot's monotone voice hums from the plane's PA system.

You immediately swing the main door shut and pull down on the handle, looking for the green light indicating that it is sealed properly. After the light illuminates, you pick up the PA microphone and say, "Ladies and gentlemen, please prepare for departure from the gate. We are expecting today's flight to LaGuardia to take about four hours and 12 minutes."

As the large aircraft rumbles backward from the steel and glass walls of the terminal, you check the overhead compartment locks one final time before strapping yourself into the aft jump seat and flipping through a magazine.

You barely notice as the jet speeds down the runway and rises steeply into the cloudy sky. You soon grow bored with the magazine—you have read it several times already—and you're looking down at the cloud layer dropping far below the window, when you sense that someone is standing over you. You look up and see a young man with panic in his face.

"Sir." You smile. "You're going to need to return to your seat until the pilot—"

"I think my girlfriend is having her baby."

"What?" You unbuckle and stand up. "Where? How do you know?"

"We're pretty sure her water broke as we took off, and now she's having a lot of contractions. She's only at 36 weeks. Please help us!"

You follow the man up the aisle to the front of the cabin, where you find a woman looking just as panicked as he does. Her face is flushed and dripping with sweat as she holds her stomach, breathing in rhythmic pants.

You hurry up to the galley, grab the medical bag, and pick up the cockpit phone, which beeps several times in your ear before you hear the co-pilot's friendly voice. "We've got a woman in labor back here," you say. "I don't think she's going to make it to LaGuardia."

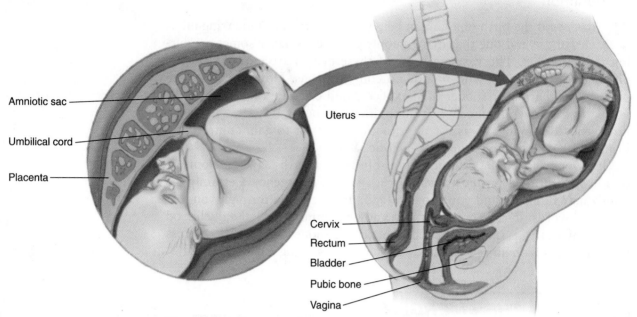

Amniotic sac
Umbilical cord
Placenta
Uterus
Cervix
Rectum
Bladder
Pubic bone
Vagina

Figure 13.1 Structures of pregnancy.

13.1 Describe the anatomy of pregnancy.

uterus the muscular organ that houses the developing fetus.

fetus a medical term that refers to the unborn child.

ovary the organ that produces the egg, or ovum.

fallopian tube the pair of tubes along which ova (eggs) travel from the ovaries to the uterus.

placenta a complex vascular organ that permits the exchange of blood and other nutrients necessary to keep the fetus alive and growing.

umbilical cord the structure that connects the fetus to the placenta.

amniotic sac the fluid-filled sac that surrounds the developing fetus.

amniotic fluid the clear, watery substance inside the amniotic sac.

13.2 Describe the three stages of labor and when each begins and ends.

trimester a period of three months; commonly used to describe the progression of a pregnancy.

THE ANATOMY OF PREGNANCY

The female body contains anatomy that is unique to the conception, development, and birth of a new life (▲ Figure 13.1). The **uterus** is the muscular organ that houses the developing **fetus** (a medical term for unborn child). The **ovary** is the organ that produces the egg, or ovum. Once released from one of the two ovaries, the egg travels through one of the two **fallopian tubes**, where it eventually is deposited into the uterus.

After the egg is fertilized, it implants on the inside wall of the uterus, where it will spend the next 40 weeks developing into a full-sized baby. As the fetus grows and develops, it is connected to the wall of the uterus by way of the **placenta**. The placenta is a complex vascular organ that permits the exchange of blood and other nutrients necessary to keep the fetus alive and growing. The fetus is connected to the placenta by way of an **umbilical cord**.

The fetus is surrounded by a thin sac called an **amniotic sac**. The sac is filled with a clear fluid, called the **amniotic fluid**, which serves to protect the developing fetus.

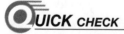 **CHECK**

Where does the fertilized egg attach itself to grow and develop for 40 weeks? ●

THE STAGES OF LABOR

The normal gestation period for a human fetus is 40 weeks. It is quite common for people to refer to this as a period of nine months, but the medical community prefers to describe the gestation process in terms of weeks. The gestation period also is broken into larger segments of three months each, called the first, second, and third **trimester**.

Labor is the process the woman's body goes through to deliver a fetus. It is characterized by gradually increasing **contractions** of the muscular uterus. The contractions cause the fetus to be pushed through the opening of the uterus, which is called the **cervix**. During labor, the cervix starts out closed and eventually opens to approximately ten centimeters to allow for the delivery of the fetus.

There are three stages of labor for a normal childbirth:

- **First stage.** Begins with the onset of regular contractions and ends with full dilation (opening) of the cervix.
- **Second stage.** Begins with the full dilation of the cervix and ends with the delivery of the baby.
- **Third stage.** Begins after the delivery of the baby and ends with the delivery of the placenta.

EVALUATING THE MOTHER

Of course, it is always best to activate your Emergency Action Plan or call 911 when faced with a woman in labor. However, sometimes a delivery will occur even before EMS arrives. So when confronted with what appears to be a pregnant woman in labor, one of the first things you must do is assess the situation to see if delivery in the field appears imminent.

Some of the questions you must ask to help you determine an **imminent birth** or the urgency of the situation are:

- **Have you been receiving prenatal care?** This question is important because it can give you a sense of whether the pregnancy has progressed normally so far. If the person has been under the care of a doctor throughout the pregnancy, she will know if things have been normal. If she has not received prenatal care, you must assume there may be complications.
- **How far along are you?** This will let you know where in the gestation process the baby and mother are. Obviously, the closer to 40 weeks, the more likely this could be a normal delivery.
- **How many children have you given birth to?** It is quite typical for each subsequent labor to be shorter than the previous one. Asking how long the woman's last labor was can help you determine the urgency of the situation.
- **Has your water broken?** This question refers to the rupturing of the amniotic sac and the rush of fluid that will occur when that happens. The amniotic sac typically will rupture within a few hours before the birth.
- **How long have you been in labor?** While each woman's labor can vary greatly from another woman's labor, an average labor takes approximately 12 hours. All things being equal, a woman who has only been in labor for three hours is less likely to deliver than a woman who has been in labor for 10 hours.
- **How far apart are your contractions?** As mentioned above, contractions are the tightening of the muscles of the uterus. Contractions occur more frequently and with greater intensity as the birth of the baby gets closer. Contractions can be hours apart when they first begin and become a minute or less apart right before delivery. The closer together they are, the more likely birth will occur.

labor the process a woman's body goes through to deliver a fetus.

contractions the shortening of the uterine muscles, which occurs at intervals before and during childbirth.

cervix the opening of the uterus.

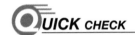

QUICK CHECK

What is labor, and how is it characterized?●

13.3 Describe the signs and symptoms of an imminent delivery.

imminent birth a situation in which the birth of a baby is highly likely to occur immediately or within minutes.

Figure 13.2 Crowning occurs when the baby's head pushes against the inside of the vaginal opening.

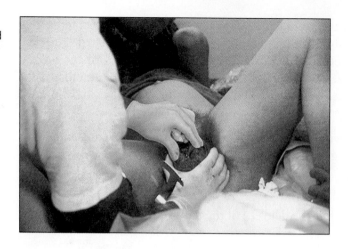

Figure 13.2 Crowning occurs when the baby's head pushes against the inside of the vaginal opening.

To determine how far apart contractions are, you must time the contraction interval. It is measured by noting the time at the beginning of a contraction and then counting the time until the beginning of the next contraction; in other words, from the beginning of one to the beginning of the next.

birth canal the interior of the vagina.

- **Do you feel the need to bear down?** When the fetus has moved out of the uterus, it enters the **birth canal**, or vagina. The vagina lies directly over the rectum. The weight of the baby pressing down on the rectum in this location causes the mother to feel as if she needs to have a bowel movement. The presence of this feeling should be assessed, because it will tell you that the baby has emerged from the uterus and has entered the birth canal.

After you have completed your questioning, it may be appropriate to conduct a visual inspection of the mother to check for evidence of crowning (▲ Figure 13.2). **Crowning** is the bulging that occurs at the opening of the vagina when the baby's head is pushing from the inside. Be sure to obtain permission from the mother and tell her exactly what you are doing and why. Ask any unnecessary bystanders to leave the scene out of respect for the mother. It is appropriate to allow the father or others close to the mother to remain with her during your inspection. If you see crowning, birth is imminent, and you should immediately prepare the scene for the delivery of the baby.

crowning the bulging that occurs at the opening of the vagina when the baby's head is pushing from the inside.

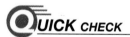 **QUICK** CHECK

What is the best way to determine the interval between contractions?

SAFETY CHECK

Due to the nature of childbirth, you are at great risk for exposure to blood and other body fluids. It is very important that you wear all appropriate personal protective equipment when assisting with a field delivery. ●

THE DELIVERY

Signs and Symptoms of an Imminent Delivery

When a delivery is imminent and there is no time to wait for EMS personnel, you must immediately prepare for the delivery of the baby at the scene. The following are some of the common signs and symptoms that a delivery may be imminent:

- Pregnancy that is full term (40 weeks)
- Contractions that are less the five minutes apart

![OB kit contents photograph]

Figure 13.3 Contents of an OB kit.

- The woman feeling the need to have a bowel movement
- Presence of crowning

Preparing for a Delivery

Once you have determined that delivery may be imminent, it is time to prepare for the delivery of the baby. There is a type of first-aid kit called an "OB kit" (▲ Figure 13.3) that contains all the tools and equipment necessary to assist with a field delivery. While an OB kit is not essential for a successful field delivery, it does make the process a little easier (Table 13.1).

13.4 Explain the steps for assisting with a field delivery.

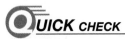UICK CHECK

What are some indications that a delivery is imminent? ●

TABLE 13.1 Contents of an OB Kit
Sterile gloves
Towels or drapes
Scissors or knife (used to cut umbilical cord)
Umbilical clamps
Gauze pads or sponges
Bulb syringe (used for suction)
Disposable blanket for baby
Sanitary napkins
Plastic bag for placenta

Assisting with the Delivery

The following steps will help guide you through the process of preparing for and assisting with a field delivery (Scan 13.1):

1. Take appropriate body substance isolation (BSI) precautions by donning gloves and eye protection, at a minimum. If available, a protective gown should be worn as well.

2. Ensure the privacy of the mother by asking nonessential people to step away from the scene.

3. Position the mother on her back with her knees bent, feet flat, and legs wide apart.

4. Place a clean drape, towel, or sheet under the mother's buttocks. Open the OB kit, if available, and ready the contents for use.

5. Position yourself between the mother's legs so you can observe the vagina and assist the baby during delivery.

6. When the baby's head begins to emerge from the vagina, apply gentle pressure with your hand against the baby's head. This is meant to help control the speed of the delivery and prevent a rapid delivery, which could be harmful to the mother. *Do not attempt to stop the delivery*. It may take several contractions before the head delivers completely.

7. Once the head has delivered, be sure to continue to support the baby's head at all times. Use the bulb syringe from the OB kit to suction out nasal or oral secretions only when they are obviously obstructing the baby's breathing.[1]

8. Next, use two fingers to feel around the baby's neck for the presence of the umbilical cord. If you feel the cord, use your fingers to slip it over the baby's head. Attempting to deliver the baby with the cord around the neck could be harmful to the baby. If the mother feels another contraction before you are done checking for a cord, instruct her to "pant" through the next contraction and not to push. Instruct her not to hold her breath but instead to take rapid, short breaths to minimize the urge to push.

9. Once you have confirmed the cord is not around the neck, be ready for the delivery of the rest of the baby. Be cautious, the baby will be very slippery. Using both hands to support the head, guide the head downward to help facilitate the delivery of the upper shoulder. Then guide the head upward for the bottom shoulder to deliver. Be ready. The baby can emerge very quickly at this point. The baby will be very slippery, so you must use both hands for support.

10. Once the baby is born quickly and thoroughly dry the baby. Once dry, wrap the baby securely in warm, dry cloths or towels. The baby should

---

[1]Kattwinkel J, Perlman JM, Aziz K, Colby C, Fairchild K, Gallagher J, Hazinski MF, Halamek LP, Kumar P, Little G, McGowan JE, Nightengale B, Ramirez MM, Ringer S, Simon WM, Weiner GM, Wyckoff M, Zaichkin J. Part 15: neonatal resuscitation: 2010 American Heart Association Guidelines for Cardiopulmonary Resuscitation and Emergency Cardiovascular Care. Circulation. 2010;122(suppl 3):S909–S919.

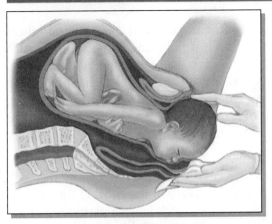

13.1.1 As the mother pushes with each contraction, support the infant's head.

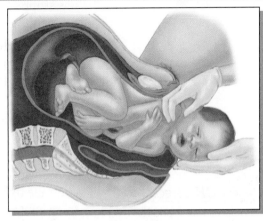

13.1.2 Once the head is delivered, check for the presence of the cord around the baby's neck.

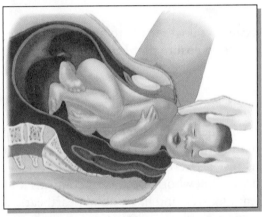

13.1.3 Next, assist with the birth of the shoulders by guiding the head downward and then upward.

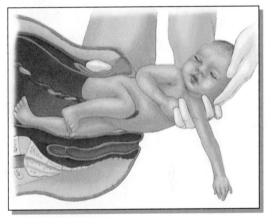

13.1.4 Be sure to support the head and torso as the body delivers.

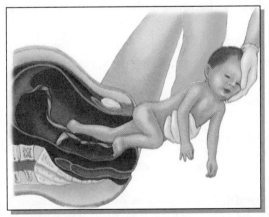

13.1.5 Use both hands, because the baby will be very slippery until dried off.

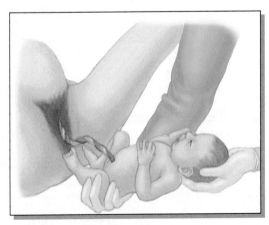

13.1.6 Keep the infant level with the vagina until the umbilical cord stops pulsating.

be crying at this point and moving good air in and out of his or her lungs. Keep the baby at or below the level of the mother's heart until the cord has stopped pulsating and is cut.

11. Once the baby is dry and warm, you can clamp and cut the umbilical cord. First, feel the cord to ensure it is not pulsating. A pulsating cord is an active cord, and you must wait for it to stop pulsating before cutting. Then place the first clamp no less than four inches from the infant. The second clamp can be placed approximately two inches from the first, away from the baby. Use a pair of clean scissors or the knife from the OB kit to cut the cord between the two clamps.

12. Place the baby on the mother's chest and allow the mother to hold the baby.

13. You must now prepare for the delivery of the placenta. The mother will continue to have contractions after the delivery of the baby. During one of these contractions, the placenta will be delivered. Have a plastic bag ready to receive the placenta. A bag is typically in the OB kit. The placenta will usually deliver within 20 to 30 minutes following the delivery of the baby.

14. Continue to monitor the ABCs (airway, breathing, circulation) of both mother and baby until EMS or other health-care providers arrive and take over care.

Your job is not complete just because you were able to assist with a successful delivery. There is still much to do to ensure that both the mother and baby are well.

Care of the Newborn

13.5 Explain the priorities of care for the infant following a field delivery.

Much like the care of a full-grown adult, the place to begin with assessing the well-being of a newborn is by evaluating the status of the ABCs. There is a good chance that the baby who has just delivered is screaming and crying. This is exactly what you want to see with a newborn, because it confirms that the airway is clear and that he is breathing well and has a good heartbeat.

Follow these steps when caring for a newborn who does not appear to have normal ABCs following delivery:

1. If the baby is unresponsive and is not breathing or only gasping, and has no pulse (or you are unsure whether there is a pulse or not), start chest compressions.

2. After 30 compressions (15 compressions if two rescuers), open the airway with a head-tilt/chin-lift and give two breaths. Use enough breath to just make the chest rise.

3. If nasal or oral secretions are obviously obstructing breathing, suction them out with a bulb syringe.[1]

4. Continue resuscitation until EMS personnel arrive. Follow infant CPR guidelines for resuscitation.

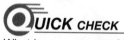

QUICK CHECK
What is your first priority following the delivery of the baby's head? ●

QUICK CHECK
What is your course of action when a newborn infant is not breathing? ●

---

[1]Kattwinkel J, Perlman JM, Aziz K, Colby C, Fairchild K, Gallagher J, Hazinski MF, Halamek LP, Kumar P, Little G, McGowan JE, Nightengale B, Ramirez MM, Ringer S, Simon WM, Weiner GM, Wyckoff M, Zaichkin J. Part 15: neonatal resuscitation: 2010 American Heart Association Guidelines for Cardiopulmonary Resuscitation and Emergency Cardiovascular Care. *Circulation*. 2010;122(suppl 3):S909–S919.

Care of the Mother

The mother has just been through a very painful event, and there is additional care and support needed to ensure that she recovers appropriately. The biggest concern for the mother following birth is blood loss. While a certain amount of blood loss during childbirth is quite normal, it is necessary to monitor blood loss because it can become life threatening.

Follow these steps when caring for a mother following childbirth:

1. Monitor the ABCs as appropriate. Keep the mother lying flat, or allow her to sit up slightly if she prefers.
2. Place a sanitary napkin or other absorbent pad over the opening of the vagina and have her keep her legs together.
3. Provide oxygen if available. Follow local protocols.
4. Monitor vital signs every 15 minutes.

If the mother has intentions of breastfeeding her baby, it is recommended to encourage the baby to nurse right away. Once you are sure that the baby is breathing adequately on his own, you may lay the baby on the mother's chest, skin to skin, and allow the baby to begin breastfeeding, if the mother is so inclined.

COMPLICATIONS RELATED TO CHILDBIRTH

There are several complications that you should be aware of during childbirth. If you encounter any of these emergencies, you must ensure that 911 has been called and that you provide the appropriate care until EMS arrives. The following emergencies pose a threat to both the mother and the baby and will not likely result in a successful field delivery. These situations require professional medical attention immediately:

- **Breech birth.** A **breech birth** occurs when the baby is not properly positioned inside the uterus during labor and presents buttocks (or limb) first instead of headfirst.
- **Prolapsed cord.** When the umbilical cord presents through the vagina before the baby's head appears, it is called a **prolapsed cord.** This is dangerous because it can cause the cord to be pinched by the baby's head during delivery. This can cause the circulation of blood and oxygen to the baby to be compromised and result in the death of the baby before delivery.
- **Severe bleeding.** There are several reasons why the mother may start bleeding severely during labor, and one of the most common is a condition known as **placenta previa.** This occurs when the placenta implants itself or grows over the opening of the cervix. When the cervix begins to dilate in anticipation of childbirth, it causes tearing of the placenta, which results in uncontrolled bleeding.

As stated previously, complications related to childbirth cannot be managed by the Emergency Responder; they require immediate medical attention. Activate your Emergency Action Plan or call 911. While you are waiting for

13.6 Explain the priorities of care for the mother following a field delivery.

13.7 Explain the common complications related to a field delivery and how to properly care for each.

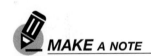

MAKE A NOTE

The vast majority of births are uneventful and will occur with or without your assistance. Your primary role is to assist the mother and help keep the situation under control.

breech birth occurs when the baby is not properly positioned inside the uterus during labor and presents buttocks (or limb) first instead of head first.

prolapsed cord occurs when the umbilical cord presents through the vagina before the baby's head crowns.

placenta previa occurs when the placenta implants itself or grows over the opening of the cervix.

Figure 13.4 Knee-chest position.

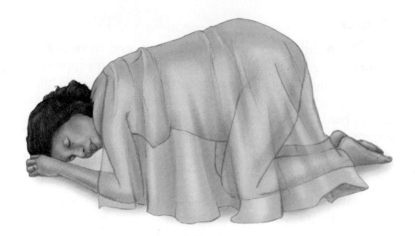

EMS or other health-care providers to arrive, follow these steps to help care for the mother and child:

1. For any severe bleeding, place a sanitary napkin or trauma dressing over the vagina and replace as often as necessary. Do not discard the used napkins or gauze pads. These will help the medical professionals evaluate the amount of blood loss. Keep the mother lying flat. Instruct her to "pant" through each contraction to minimize the urge to push during a contraction.

2. In the instance of a breech presentation or a prolapsed cord, place the mother in a knee-chest position (▲ Figure 13.4). Place a pillow under her head and instruct her to pant through each contraction to minimize the urge to push during contractions.

3. Provide supplemental oxygen if available. Follow local protocols.

4. Monitor vital signs every five minutes.

MAKE A NOTE

It is important to ask the mother if she knows that she is carrying only one baby or if she is carrying twins or triplets. There is nothing you need to do to prepare for multiple births except gather additional blankets and towels for receiving the babies and for keeping them dry and warm. Most OB kits have four clamps for just such an event. ●

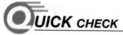UICK CHECK

How does asking a mother to pant through a contraction help during a complicated delivery such as a prolapsed cord? ●

THE HANDOFF

You cleared the row, repositioning passengers to several vacant seats so the woman could lie on her back. As the jet begins the final approach after circling back and returning to the original airport, you check visually and find that the baby is crowning.

"I need to push," the panting woman nearly shouts.

"That's fine," you say, putting gentle pressure on the top of the baby's head with your gloved hand. "If you need to push, then push. I'm going to help you through this."

The aircraft touches down smoothly, slows to a taxi, and heads immediately to gate 19 where an ambulance crew is waiting to board. Once the concourse has been positioned, one of your coworkers pops the door and two EMTs clamber aboard, carrying equipment bags and an oxygen cylinder.

"Looks like you did a great job," one of the EMTs says to you, seeing that the newborn is wrapped in a blanket and lying on the smiling mother's stomach.

"I didn't do anything with the cord," you say, wiping the sweat off of your forehead with the back of your hand.

"That's fine." The EMT smiles. "You did exactly what you were supposed to do."

"Thank you so much." The new mother grabs your hand as the EMTs are rolling her out of the plane in a wheelchair. "I'm sorry I messed up the flight for everyone."

"Don't worry about it," you say, patting her arm. "Of all the reasons for a flight delay, this is one I definitely don't mind."

CHAPTER REVIEW

Chapter Summary

- Some anatomical structures are unique to women. They support the conception and development of a fetus. Those structures are the ovaries, where the eggs are made; the fallopian tubes, which connect the ovaries to the uterus; and the uterus, which serves as the home for the fetus during development.

- Labor is the process that the woman's body goes through to deliver a baby. There are three stages of labor. The first stage begins with the onset of contractions and ends with full dilation of the cervix. The second stage begins with full dilation of the cervix and ends with the birth of the baby. The third stage includes the delivery of the placenta.

- There are several signs and symptoms that will tell you that a birth is imminent: a pregnancy that is full term (40 weeks), contractions that are less the five minutes apart, the woman feeling the need to have a bowel movement, and the presence of crowning.

- Your job is to assist the mother with the delivery of the baby by preparing the scene for the delivery, assisting with the delivery, ensuring that the baby is breathing well and has good circulation, and assisting with the delivery of the placenta.

- Just because you have successfully delivered a baby does not mean the work is over. You must continue to closely monitor the baby's ABCs to ensure that he or she is breathing properly and has good circulation. If not, you must provide rescue breaths or begin CPR as appropriate.

- The care of the mother does not end following delivery of the baby. You must monitor the mother for excessive bleeding and monitor vital signs until EMS personnel arrives and takes over care.

- There are some complications that can arise during delivery. Excessive bleeding could be caused by a condition known as placenta previa and requires immediate attention by EMS personnel. A breech presentation is one where the baby attempts to deliver buttocks or limbs first, and a prolapsed cord occurs when the umbilical cord presents before the baby does. Those situations require professional medical care. Position the mother in a knee-chest position and instruct her to pant through each contraction until EMS or other health-care providers arrive.

Quick Quiz

1. When the umbilical cord protrudes from the vagina prior to delivery of the baby, it is called a _____ cord.
   a. premature
   b. prolapsed
   c. crowning
   d. ruptured

2. Which one of the following questions would NOT be appropriate to ask a woman who is in active labor?
   a. Has your water broken?
   b. Have you been seeing a doctor for your pregnancy?
   c. How many children have you given birth to?
   d. How old were you when you became sexually active?

3. You are caring for a woman who is in labor, and you can see that the baby's head is crowning. How would you help prevent a too rapid delivery?
   a. Ask her to close her legs.
   b. Have her get on all fours and keep her back arched.
   c. Place gentle pressure on the baby's head with your gloved hand.
   d. Instruct her not to push with the contractions.

4. Which stage of labor actually begins after the baby is born?
   a. First
   b. Second
   c. Third
   d. Fourth

5. Under normal circumstances, the placenta will deliver within about _____ after the birth of the baby.
   a. 20 to 30 minutes
   b. 5 to 10 minutes
   c. 1 to 2 hours
   d. 40 to 60 minutes

6. A young woman gives birth to a baby boy that is calm, quiet, and seems to be staring at the lights above you. You should:
   a. wrap the baby in a warm blanket and place him on his mother's stomach.
   b. provide several rescue breaths, being careful not to overinflate his lungs.
   c. cut the umbilical cord and use a basin to give the baby a warm bath.
   d. flick his feet or rub his skin with a towel.

7. A coworker tells you that she is in labor, has already called 911, and needs your help to possibly deliver the baby. While preparing her, you notice that the baby's leg is protruding from the vagina. You should immediately:
   a. realize that the baby is in a breech presentation and attempt to push the leg back in.
   b. move the woman into a knee-chest position and instruct her to pant through each contraction until the ambulance arrives.
   c. grasp the leg and gently but steadily pull the baby out, ensuring that the umbilical cord does not wrap around the baby's neck.
   d. roll the woman into the recovery position and instruct her to squeeze her legs together.

8. You are called to assist a woman in her 39th week of pregnancy. She has been complaining of strong, frequent contractions and immediately asks you to help her to the bathroom because she feels the need to have a bowel movement. How might you determine if the birth is imminent?
   a. Feel for the presence of crowning.
   b. Encourage her to use the bathroom.
   c. Observe for crowning.
   d. Feel her stomach to determine the intensity of the contractions.

Appendix 1

Blood Pressure Monitoring

LEARNING OBJECTIVES

At the conclusion of this appendix and the associated instructor-guided lesson, the student will be able to:

Cognitive

A1.1 Explain the relationship between blood pressure and circulation. *(p. 185)*

A1.2 Identify the parts of a blood pressure cuff. *(p. 186)*

A1.3 State why palpation might be used instead of auscultation when obtaining a blood pressure. *(p. 190)*

Psychomotor

A1.4 Demonstrate the ability to accurately auscultate a blood pressure.

A1.5 Demonstrate the ability to accurately palpate a blood pressure.

KEY TERMS

The following terms are introduced in this appendix:

- auscultation *(p. 187)*
- blood pressure *(p. 185)*
- diastolic pressure *(p. 186)*
- palpation *(p. 187)*
- sphygmomanometer *(p. 186)*
- stethoscope *(p. 187)*
- systolic pressure *(p. 186)*

Introduction

As you already learned in Chapter 7, there are specific characteristics that you can identify and measure called vital signs. Vital signs are called that because they are vital to a person's well-being and strong indicators of the status of the ill or injured person. Chapter 7 addressed respirations, pulse, and skin signs. Another important vital sign that requires specialized equipment and training to obtain is called blood pressure. This appendix explains what blood pressure is and introduces you to the proper technique for obtaining a blood pressure measurement.

In some localities, particularly those in which Emergency Responders work in isolated areas, special training for learning to assess blood pressure may be desired or required.

WHAT IS BLOOD PRESSURE?

Blood pressure is the measurement of the pressure of blood against the inside of the walls of the arteries. Blood pressure is an essential element of good circulation. When blood pressure is normal, it ensures that blood is being circulated to all of the cells of the body. A blood pressure reading that is significantly above or below the normal range for a person can be a

A1.1 Explain the relationship between blood pressure and circulation.

blood pressure the measurement of the pressure of blood against the inside of the walls of the arteries.

185

valuable tool in determining the current state or condition of the ill or injured person.

Blood pressure is determined by measuring the pressure changes in the arteries. When the heart contracts, it forces blood into the aorta and other arteries to circulate throughout the body. The pressure generated in the arteries when the heart contracts is called the systolic blood pressure. The **systolic pressure** is affected by many factors, such as the force of the heart's pumping action and blood volume within the body. (Blood loss means lower pressure.)

After each contraction of the heart, it relaxes and refills. This relaxation phase is called diastole. During diastole, the pressure in the arteries falls. When measured, this pressure is called the **diastolic pressure**.

Blood pressure is measured using a device called a **sphygmomanometer**, or, more simply, a blood pressure cuff. A blood pressure cuff is made up of a flat rubber balloon called a bladder that is contained within a cloth pouch called a cuff. Leading from the bladder are two tubes. One tube is connected to an inflation bulb and valve. The other is connected to a gauge used to measure the blood pressure readings. The gauge is calibrated in specific units called millimeters of mercury (mm Hg). Since this system of measurement is standard, you will not have to say "millimeters of mercury" after each reading. Report the systolic pressure first and then the diastolic, as in 120 over 80 (120/80).

The reading of 120/80 or lower is considered a normal blood pressure reading, which represents the average blood pressure obtained from a large sampling of healthy adults. There is a wide range of "normal" for adults and children. You will not know the normal blood pressure for any individual unless he is alert, knows the information, and can tell you what it is. It is a good practice to always ask the person if he knows what his blood pressure normally is prior to taking it yourself. Knowing this will help you determine if the reading that you get is normal for him.

A systolic blood pressure reading below 90 mm Hg is considered lower than normal in most adults. However, some small adult females and small-build athletes may have a normal systolic blood pressure of 90 mm Hg or lower. A systolic reading above 140 is typically considered high blood pressure, also referred to as hypertension. Many ill or injured people will show an initial rise in blood pressure at the emergency scene. This is usually due to anxiety, fear, or stress caused by the incident and will return to normal once the situation or condition is under control.

Determining accurate blood pressures requires a fair amount of practice. Practice this skill frequently. Establishing a trend in blood pressure (going up, going down, staying the same) is more important than the absolute value of the blood pressure in the emergency care setting.[1]

---

[1]T. G. Pickering et al., " Recommendations for Blood Pressure Measurement in Humans and Experimental Animals, Part 1: Blood Pressure Measurement in Humans: A Statement for Professionals from the Subcommittee of Professional and Public Education of the American Heart Association Council on High Blood Pressure Research," *Circulation* 111 (2005): 697–716, http://circ.ahajournals.org/cgi/content/full/111/5/697 (accessed January 13, 2010).

Guidelines for blood pressure readings are as follows:

Adults

- Systolic above 140 is borderline high.
- Systolic below 80 is borderline low (although it depends on size and age of the person).
- Diastolic above 90 is borderline high.

Children: Ages 6 to 14

- Systolic above 140 is borderline high.
- Systolic below 80 is borderline low.
- Diastolic above 70 is borderline high.

MEASURING BLOOD PRESSURE

There are two common techniques used to measure blood pressure in emergency care. The first is by listening, which is called **auscultation**, and it requires the use of a **stethoscope**. The second is by feeling, which is called **palpation**. The palpation method will only reveal the systolic pressure.

auscultation taking a blood pressure reading by listening through a stethoscope.

stethoscope an instrument used for listening to sounds within the body.

palpation taking a blood pressure reading by feeling the pulse with the fingertips.

Determining Blood Pressure by Auscultation

The auscultation method requires the use of a stethoscope to hear the sound of the blood pulsating through the artery. You must begin by adjusting the earpieces so that they fit properly in your ears. Hold the earpieces of the stethoscope between the thumb and index finger of each hand. Adjust the direction of the earpieces by gently turning them so that each piece points slightly forward (away from you). This is to ensure that the openings of the earpieces point directly into your ear canals when placed in the ears and will help ensure that you will hear the pulsations once the bladder is inflated.

To determine blood pressure using a blood pressure cuff and a stethoscope, you should (Scans A1.1, A1.2, and A1.3):

1. Have the ill or injured person sit or lie down. Cut away or remove clothing that is on the arm. Support the arm at the level of the heart. Do not use the person's arm if there is any possibility of injury.
2. Select the correct-size blood pressure cuff. The average adult cuff can accommodate an arm that is up to 13 inches in circumference.
3. Wrap the cuff around the person's upper arm. The lower border of the cuff should be about one inch above the crease in the elbow. The center of the bladder inside the cuff must be placed over the brachial artery in the upper arm.

   Some cuffs have a marker to indicate how to line up the cuff over the brachial artery. Some cuffs have no markers, while others have inaccurate markers. Locate the center of the bladder and line it up over the brachial artery on the inside of the arm.
4. Apply the cuff securely but not too tightly. You should be able to place one finger under the bottom edge of the cuff.

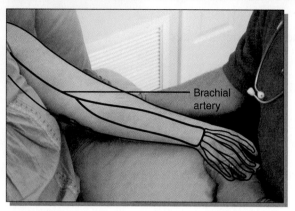

A1.1.1 Have the person sit or lie down. Support the arm so that it is extended. Note the location of the brachial artery.

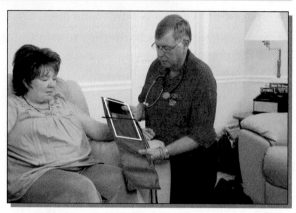

A1.1.2 Select an appropriate size blood pressure cuff. Locate the center of the bladder inside the cuff.

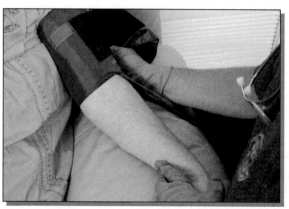

A1.1.3 Place the cuff firmly around the upper arm, making sure the center of the bladder is over the brachial artery on the inside of the arm.

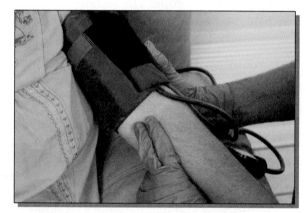

A1.1.4 Locate the brachial pulse point at the anterior side of the elbow. This will be where you place your stethoscope.

5. Place the ends of the stethoscope in your ears. Be sure to adjust the earpieces so that they face forward into your ear canals. They are easily adjustable. If you are using a dual-head stethoscope, make certain to check that the appropriate side is activated before placing it.

6. Use your fingertips to locate the brachial artery at the crease in the elbow.

7. Position the diaphragm of the stethoscope over the brachial artery pulse site. Do not let the head of the stethoscope touch the cuff. If it touches the cuff, the stethoscope will rub against it during inflation and deflation. You will hear the rubbing sounds, which may cause you to record a false reading.

8. Close the valve and inflate the cuff to approximately 180 mm Hg for an adult and 120 mm Hg for a child. Place your fingertips over the radial pulse as you inflate the cuff. When you can no longer feel the pulse,

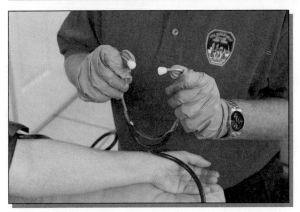

A1.2.1 Before placing the stethoscope in your ears, make certain that the earpieces are adjusted properly. They must point slightly forward (away from you).

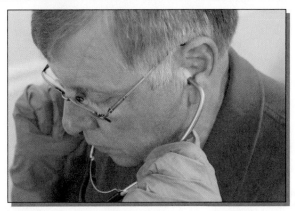

A1.2.2 Carefully place the stethoscope in your ears.

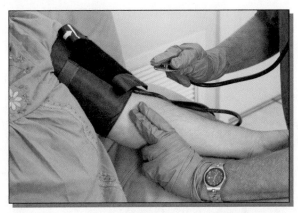

A1.2.3 Next, place the diaphragm of the stethoscope over the brachial pulse point that you identified earlier.

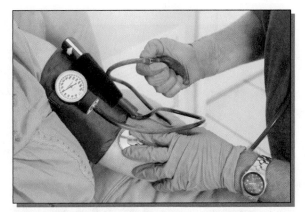

A1.2.4 Inflate and deflate the cuff as appropriate to determine the blood pressure.

pump up the cuff pressure 30 more mm Hg. Then slowly release the pressure as you listen for the pulse sounds.

9. Once the cuff is inflated, open the valve slowly to release pressure from the cuff. It should fall at a smooth rate of 2 to 3 mm Hg per second or a little faster than the second hand on a watch.

10. Listen carefully as you watch the needle move. Note when you hear the sound of the pulse in the stethoscope. The first significant sound that you hear is the systolic pressure.

11. Let the cuff continue to deflate. Listen for and note when the sound of the pulse (clicking or tapping) fades (not when it stops). When the sound turns dull or soft, this is the diastolic pressure.

12. Let the rest of the air out of the cuff quickly. If practical, leave the cuff in place so you can take additional readings. Be sure to squeeze the cuff to release all the air.

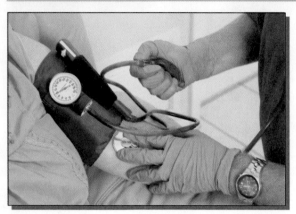

A1.3.1 With the stethoscope in place, briskly inflate the cuff.

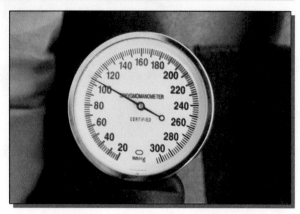

A1.3.2 Deflate the cuff slowly while watching the gauge and listening with the stethoscope. Note where the needle is for the first sound you hear (systolic) and the last sound you hear (diastolic).

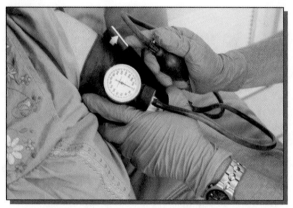

A1.3.3 When you are done taking the blood pressure, squeeze the cuff to force out any remaining air pressure.

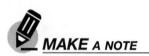

MAKE A NOTE

The average adult cuff can accommodate an arm that is up to 13 inches in circumference. A cuff that is too small will produce falsely high readings, and one that is too large will produce falsely low readings. ●

A1.3 State why palpation might be used instead of auscultation when obtaining a blood pressure.

13. Record the time, the arm used, the position of the ill or injured person (lying down, sitting), and the pressure readings. Round off the readings to the next highest number. For example, 145 mm Hg should be recorded as 146 mm Hg. (The markings on the gauge are in even numbers. You may "see" the first sound in between two markings and want to record it as an odd number—145—but all blood pressure readings are recorded in even numbers.)

If you are not certain of a reading, be sure the cuff is totally deflated and wait one or two minutes and try again, or use the person's other arm. Should you try the same arm too soon, you may get a false high reading.

Determining Blood Pressure by Palpation

Using the palpation method (feeling the radial pulse) is not a very accurate method. It will provide you with one reading—an approximate systolic pressure. This method is used when there is too much ambient noise, making it difficult to hear with a stethoscope.

To determine blood pressure by palpation, place the cuff in the same position on the arm as you would for auscultation. Then proceed with the following:

1. Find the radial pulse on the arm with the cuff.
2. Close the valve and inflate the cuff until you can no longer feel the pulse.
3. Continue to inflate the cuff to a point 30 mm Hg above the point where the pulse disappeared.
4. Slowly deflate the cuff and note the reading when you feel the pulse return. This is the systolic blood pressure. You will not get a diastolic pressure reading by palpation.
5. Record the time, the arm used, the position of the person, and the systolic pressure. Note that the reading was by palpation. If you give this information orally to someone, make sure they know the reading was by palpation, as in, "Blood pressure is 146 by palpation."

Appendix 2

Airway Adjuncts, Suctioning, and Oxygen Therapy

LEARNING OBJECTIVES

At the conclusion of this appendix and the associated instructor-guided lesson, the student will be able to:

Cognitive

A2.1 State the oxygen concentration of room air. *(p. 194)*

A2.2 Describe the purpose and functions of an oxygen regulator. *(p. 195)*

A2.3 Differentiate among the common sizes of oxygen cylinders. *(p. 194)*

A2.4 Explain the potential hazards of working with high-pressure cylinders. *(p. 194)*

A2.5 Explain the indications for the use of a nasal cannula. *(p. 198)*

A2.6 Explain the indications for the use of a nonrebreather mask. *(p. 200)*

A2.7 Explain the indications and contraindication for the insertion of an oropharyngeal airway. *(p. 203)*

A2.8 Explain the indications for oral suctioning. *(p. 205)*

Psychomotor

A2.9 Demonstrate the proper use of a bag-mask device.

A2.10 Demonstrate the technique for attaching a regulator to a cylinder.

A2.11 Demonstrate the use of a nasal cannula.

A2.12 Demonstrate the use of a nonrebreather mask.

A2.13 Demonstrate the use of an oropharyngeal airway (OPA).

A2.14 Demonstrate the technique for oral suctioning.

A2.15 Demonstrate the technique for nasal suctioning.

Introduction

DEPENDING on the agency or institution that you will be serving as an Emergency Responder, you may be trained in the use of additional skills. This appendix introduces the skill of administering supplemental oxygen. In addition, you will be introduced to the skills related to the insertion of basic airway adjuncts, the use of the bag-mask device, and suctioning. These skills require additional time and practice to develop proficiency. In addition to the information provided here, your instructor will facilitate classroom time when you can practice these new and important skills.

According to an evidence-based review of the scientific literature in first aid, there is no evidence for or against the routine use of oxygen as a first aid measure for victims experiencing shortness of breath or chest pain. However, the use of oxygen in first aid for recreational SCUBA divers with a decompression injury resulted in a greater likelihood of complete recovery.[1]

EMERGENCY OXYGEN

It may sound strange, but oxygen used for medical therapy is a closely regulated prescription drug. There has been some confusion about the regulations concerning the use of emergency oxygen for individuals who do not work in the health-care field, including Emergency Response Teams in business and industry. All oxygen cylinders are filled with what is known as "medical-grade" oxygen. The type of equipment that is attached to the cylinder and the intended use determines any restrictions or prescription requirements.

The following is a list of requirements pertaining to the use of oxygen for emergency care:

- It must be contained in a portable cylinder with a regulator that provides oxygen for a minimum of 15 minutes.
- The device has a constant fixed flow rate of not less than six liters per minute (LPM).
- A content indicator gauge is present to determine how much oxygen is in the cylinder.
- The device is labeled "Emergency" and has emergency operation instructions.
- A mask with a connection for oxygen tubing is supplied for oxygen administration.

If oxygen equipment is not intended for emergency use and is capable of providing less than six liters/minute, it requires a physician's prescription for use in medical applications, such as for people with chronic lung disease or other conditions that require a varied flow and dosage of oxygen supply under the direction of a medical professional. The physician's staff or other personnel (such as EMS providers) may administer it as prescribed by the physician.

Oxygen for medical use has a flow rate of 0 to 25 liters per minute that is controlled at the discretion of the operator. In September 1996, the U.S. Food and Drug Administration (FDA), the regulatory agency for medical gases, determined that labeling for all oxygen equipment would bear the following statement:

"For emergency use only when administered by properly trained personnel for oxygen deficiency and resuscitation. For all other medical applications, CAUTION: Federal law prohibits dispensing without prescription."

---

[1]Markenson D, Ferguson JD, Chameides L, Cassan P, Chung K-L, Epstein JL, Gonzales L, Hazinski MF, Herrington RA, Pellegrino JL, Ratcliff N, Singer AJ; on behalf of the First Aid Chapter Collaborators. Part 13: first aid: 2010 American Heart Association and American Red Cross International Consensus on First Aid Science. *Circulation*. 2010;122(suppl 2):S582–S605.

Even though the regulations at the federal level in the United States allow the use of emergency oxygen without a prescription, your local requirements may vary. Check the regulations that govern oxygen equipment or utilization in your location. Agencies and institutions that allow Emergency Responders to administer oxygen for medical applications must have a physician who has prescribed its use and who should assist in the development of training and protocols (guidelines) that the Emergency Responder must follow. In general, these protocols should direct that supplemental oxygen be given with a bag-mask device during two-rescuer CPR or with a nonrebreather delivery device when signs and symptoms of breathlessness, heart failure, stroke, or shock are present.[2] Your instructor should be familiar with any physican-directed protocols and be able to provide additional guidance.

A2.1 State the oxygen concentration of room air.

Hazards of Oxygen

A2.4 Explain the potential hazards of working with high-pressure cylinders.

There are certain hazards associated with oxygen administration, including:

- Oxygen used in emergency care is stored under pressure—2,000 pounds per square inch (psi) or greater. If the tank is punctured or if a valve breaks off, the supply tank and the valve can become missiles.
- Oxygen supports combustion and causes fire to burn more rapidly. Oxygen can saturate linens and clothing and cause them to ignite quickly.
- Under pressure, oxygen and oil do not mix. When they come into contact with each other, there can be a severe reaction, which may cause an explosion. This easily can occur if you try to lubricate a delivery system or gauge with petroleum products.
- Long-term use of high oxygen concentrations can result in medical dangers. These dangers include lung tissue destruction (oxygen toxicity), seizure, lung collapse, and eye damage in premature infants.

Equipment and Supplies for Oxygen Therapy

An oxygen delivery system includes several components, including a source (oxygen cylinder), pressure regulator, flow meter, and a delivery device (facemask or cannula).

Oxygen Cylinders

A2.3 Differentiate among the common sizes of oxygen cylinders.

When providing oxygen in the field, the standard source of oxygen is a seamless steel or aluminum cylinder filled with pressurized oxygen. When the cylinder is full, the pressure is approximately 2,000 psi. Cylinders come in various

---

[2]Berg RA, Hemphill R, Abella BS, Aufderheide TP, Cave DM, Hazinski MF, Lerner EB, Rea TD, Sayre MR, Swor RA. Part 5: Adult basic life support: 2010 American Heart Association Guidelines for Cardiopulmonary Resuscitation and Emergency Cardiovascular Care. *Circulation*. 2010;122(suppl 3):S685–S705.

sizes, identified by letters. The smaller sizes commonly found in the field setting are:

- D cylinder, which contains about 425 liters of oxygen.
- Jumbo D cylinder, which contains about 640 liters of oxygen.
- E cylinder, which contains about 680 liters of oxygen.

Part of your duty as an Emergency Responder is to make certain that the oxygen cylinders are full and ready for use before they are needed. In most cases you will use a pressure gauge to determine the pressure remaining in the tank. The length of time that you can use an oxygen cylinder depends on the pressure in the cylinder and the flow rate.

Oxygen cylinders should never be allowed to empty below the safe residual level. The safe residual level for an oxygen cylinder is determined when the pressure gauge reads 200 psi. (You cannot tell if an oxygen cylinder is full, partially full, or empty by lifting or moving the cylinder.) At this point, you must switch to a fresh cylinder; below this point, there is not enough oxygen for proper delivery to the person.

Safety is of prime importance when working with oxygen cylinders, so you should:

- Never allow a cylinder to drop or fall against any object. The cylinder must be well secured, preferably in a lying-down position. Never let a cylinder stand by itself.
- Never allow smoking around oxygen equipment or use around open flames or sparks.
- Never use grease or oil on devices that will be attached to an oxygen supply cylinder.
- Never store a cylinder near high heat or in a closed vehicle that is parked in the sun.
- Always use the pressure gauges and regulators that are intended for use with oxygen and the equipment you are using.

The U.S. Department of Transportation requires that all compressed gas cylinders be inspected and pressure tested at specific intervals. The cylinders that contain medical-grade oxygen must be tested every five years. This test is commonly referred to as a hydrostatic test, because following visual inspection, the tank is filled with water and pressurized to five-thirds the service pressure, or approximately 3,360 psi, to confirm that no leaks exist. The most recent hydrostatic test date must be stamped into the crown of the cylinder and easily readable.

Pressure Regulators

The pressure in an oxygen cylinder is too high to be used directly from the cylinder. A **pressure regulator** must be connected to the oxygen cylinder before it may be used to deliver oxygen to an ill or injured person. The safe working pressure for oxygen administration is 30 to 70 psi. The pressure regulator will reduce the pressure in the tank from 2,000 to a working pressure between 30 and 70 psi.

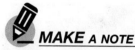
MAKE A NOTE

Some oxygen cylinders have met rigorous inspection and testing standards and are allowed to go up to 10 years between test dates. These cylinders have a five-pointed star immediately following the hydrostatic test date stamped into the crown. ●

A2.2 Describe the purpose and functions of an oxygen regulator.

pressure regulator a device used to reduce the pressure of a gas (oxygen) so that it can be easily controlled and delivered to an ill or injured person.

On cylinders of the E size or smaller, a yoke assembly is used to secure the pressure regulator to the cylinder valve assembly. The yoke has pins that must mate with the corresponding holes found in the valve assembly. This is called a pin-index safety system. The position of the pins varies for different gases to prevent an oxygen delivery system from being connected to a cylinder containing another gas.

Follow these steps to properly attach a pressure regulator to an oxygen cylinder (Scan A2.1):

1. Remove the protective seal over the cylinder valve.
2. Inspect the valve for cleanliness.
3. Quickly open and shut the cylinder valve to expel any particles of dust or debris. (This is called "cracking" the cylinder valve.)
4. Confirm the presence of an O ring, and slip the yoke of the pressure regulator over the cylinder valve.

SCAN A2.1   Attaching Regulator to Tank

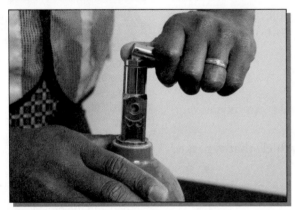

A2.1.1 Quickly open and then shut ("crack") the cylinder valve to expel dirt.

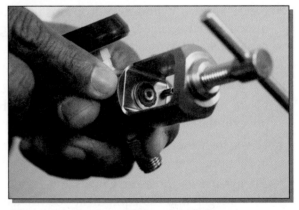

A2.1.2 Confirm the presence of an O ring.

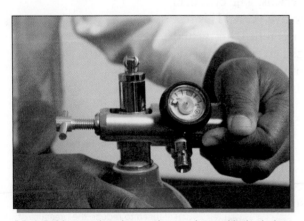

A2.1.3 Line up the pins on the regulator with the holes on the valve.

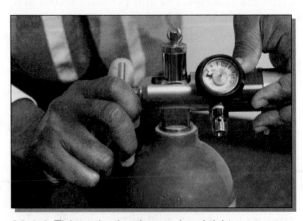

A2.1.4 Tighten the thumbscrew hand-tight.

5. Line up the pins on the regulator with the holes on the valve, and tighten the thumbscrew hand-tight.

6. Turn the pressure gauge away from you or others, and open the valve one full turn (counterclockwise).

7. Read the pressure gauge, and confirm the pressure in the cylinder.

Note that the FDA has received over a dozen reports in which regulators used with oxygen cylinders have burned or exploded, in some cases injuring personnel. The FDA and the National Institute for Occupational Safety and Health (NIOSH) believe that improper use of plastic gaskets/washers was a major factor in both the ignition and severity of the fires. The FDA and NIOSH recommend that the plastic crush gaskets commonly used to create the seal at the cylinder valve/regulator interface *never* be reused.[3]

Flowmeters

A flowmeter is connected to the pressure regulator to provide control over the flow of oxygen in liters per minute (LPM). The constant-flow selector valve is one of the most common used in the field today.

The constant-flow selector valve has no liter flow gauge. It allows for the adjustment of flow in LPM in stepped increments (2, 4, 6, 8, . . . 15 LPM). When using this type of flowmeter, make certain that it is properly adjusted for the desired flow. Monitor the dial to make certain that it stays properly adjusted.

A fixed flow regulator is required for use with emergency oxygen. Depending on the setting (6 or 12 LPM), such a system delivers a fixed flow of oxygen at a precise rate that cannot be adjusted. The oxygen flows at the fixed rate until it is turned off.

Oxygen Delivery Devices for the Breathing Person

Several types of oxygen delivery masks are available. You must become familiar with and recognize the various types so that you can choose the delivery mask appropriate for your level of training and the condition of the ill or injured person. The nasal cannula and the nonrebreather mask are the main oxygen delivery devices used for the field administration of oxygen to ill or injured people who are breathing on their own.

One of the most commonly used devices for the delivery of emergency oxygen is a barrier mask with oxygen inlet and one-way valve. A barrier mask is the same one that you use for CPR, but it is fitted with a port or inlet to which the oxygen tubing attaches (▼ Figure A2.1). It is the ideal mask to deliver emergency oxygen to either a breathing or nonbreathing victim. Sold under many brand names, this mask is the one to consider for all emergency oxygen administration.

---

[3]U.S. Food and Drug Administration, *FDA and NIOSH Public Health Notification: Oxygen Regulator Fires Resulting from Incorrect Use of CGA 870 Seals* (Silver Spring, MD: U.S. FDA, June 2006), http://www.fda.gov/MedicalDevices/Safety/AlertsandNotices/PublicHealthNotifications/ucm062088.htm (accessed January 13, 2010).

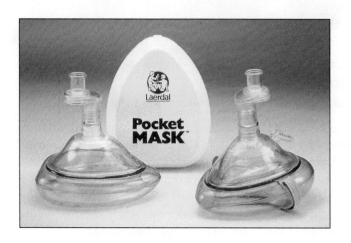

Figure A2.1 Pocket mask with one-way valve and oxygen connection. (© Laerdal Medical Corporation)

Nasal Cannula

The **nasal cannula** delivers oxygen into the person's nostrils by way of two small plastic prongs. Its efficiency is greatly reduced by nasal injuries, colds, and other types of nasal airway obstruction. A flow rate of 1 to 6 LPM will provide the person with 25–45 percent oxygen. The approximate relationship of oxygen concentration to LPM flow is as follows:

A2.5 Explain the indications for the use of a nasal cannula.

nasal cannula a device that delivers oxygen into the person's nostrils by way of two small plastic prongs.

1 LPM – 25% oxygen

2 LPM – 29% oxygen

3 LPM – 33% oxygen

4 LPM – 37% oxygen

5 LPM – 41% oxygen

6 LPM – 45% oxygen

For every 1 LPM increase in oxygen flow, you deliver a 4 percent increase in the concentration of oxygen. At 4 LPM and above, the person's breathing patterns may prevent the delivery of the stated percentages. At 5 LPM, rapid drying of the nasal membranes is possible. After 6 LPM, the device does not deliver any higher concentration of oxygen and may be uncomfortable for most people.

Follow these steps to properly apply a nasal cannula (Scan A2.2):

1. Confirm that the person is breathing with an adequate rate and tidal volume.

2. Advise the person that you are going to give him some oxygen.

3. Select the appropriate size cannula.

4. Connect the cannula supply tubing to an appropriate oxygen source, and adjust the liter flow to between 2 and 6 LPM.

5. Slide the adjusting band downward to allow for full expansion of the cannula loop.

6. Grasp the loop with the thumb and index finger of each hand on either side of the prongs.

7. Advise the person that the prongs will tickle a little bit but will not hurt. Insert the prongs into the person's nostrils.

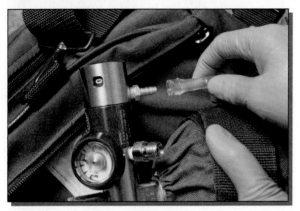

A2.2.1 Connect tube to regulator.

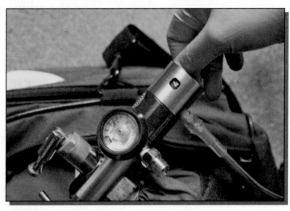

A2.2.2 Adjust liter flow.

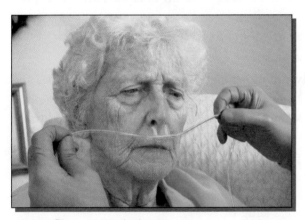

A2.2.3 Place prongs in the nose.

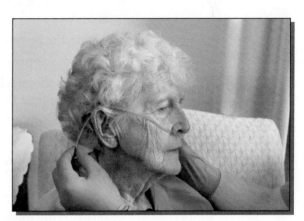

A2.2.4 Wrap tubing around ears.

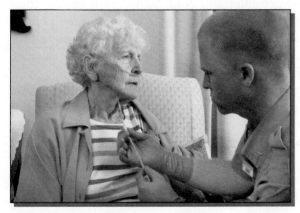

A2.2.5 Secure slide adjustor under chin.

8. Slide your fingers along the loop, and wrap each side around the person's ears.

9. Slide the adjusting band up under the chin to take up any slack in the loop. Advise the person to breathe through his nose.

A2.6 Explain the indications for the use of a nonrebreather mask.

Nonrebreather Mask

A **nonrebreather mask** is used to deliver high concentrations of oxygen. It is important that you inflate the reservoir bag before placing the mask on the person's face. This is done by using your finger to cover the one-way valve inside the mask between the mask and the reservoir. Care must be taken to ensure a proper seal with the person's face. The reservoir must not deflate by more than one-third when the person takes his deepest inhalation. You can maintain the volume in the bag by adjusting the oxygen flow. The person's exhaled air does not return to the reservoir; instead, it is vented through the one-way flaps or portholes on the mask. The minimum flow rate when using this mask is 8 LPM, but a higher flow (12–15 LPM) may be required.

nonrebreather mask a device consisting of a facemask with a one-way valve and a reservoir bag; used to deliver high concentrations of oxygen.

Follow these steps to properly apply a nonrebreather mask (Scan A2.3):

1. Confirm that the person is breathing with an adequate rate and tidal volume.

2. Advise the person that you are going to give him some oxygen.

3. Select the appropriate size mask.

4. Connect the mask supply tubing to an appropriate oxygen source, and adjust the liter flow to 15 LPM.

5. Place your thumb over the one-way valve inside the mask to expedite the filling of the reservoir.

6. Place the mask over the person's face, starting at the bridge of the nose and "walking" the mask down the face.

7. Place the elastic band around the person's head, and pull the ends through the mask to ensure a snug fit.

8. Squeeze the aluminum nose strap to help seal the mask across the nose.

Administration of Oxygen to a Nonbreathing Person

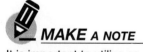

MAKE A NOTE

It is important to utilize an appropriate airway adjunct whenever possible when providing rescue breaths for a nonbreathing patient. Airway adjuncts will be discussed a little later in this appendix. ●

bag-mask device a device used to provide rescue breaths for a person with inadequate respirations; it consists of a bag, one-way-valve, and facemask.

The pocket facemask with oxygen inlet and your own breath can be combined to deliver oxygen-enriched rescue breaths to a nonbreathing person. The **bag-mask device**, alone or with 100 percent oxygen, can be used to provide rescue breaths for the nonbreathing person. When using these devices, an oropharyngeal airway (OPA) should be inserted.

Most bag-mask devices are capable of accepting supplemental oxygen. When available, attach it to an oxygen source and adjust the flow to no less than 10 to 12 LPM.[4] Many bag-mask devices have an oxygen reservoir (long tube or bag) to increase the oxygen concentration delivered. Used without a

[4]Berg RA, Hemphill R, Abella BS, Aufderheide TP, Cave DM, Hazinski MF, Lerner EB, Rea TD, Sayre MR, Swor RA. Part 5: Adult basic life support: 2010 American Heart Association Guidelines for Cardiopulmonary Resuscitation and Emergency Cardiovascular Care. *Circulation.* 2010;122(suppl 3):S685–S705.

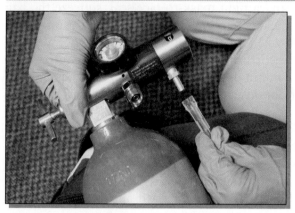

A2.3.1 Connect the mask supply tubing to an appropriate oxygen source.

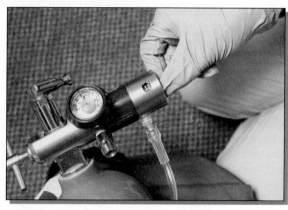

A2.3.2 Adjust the liter flow to 15 LPM.

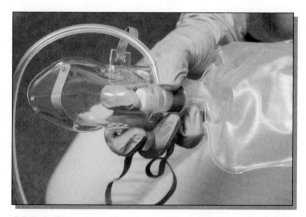

A2.3.3 Place your thumb over the one-way valve inside the mask to expedite the filling of the reservoir.

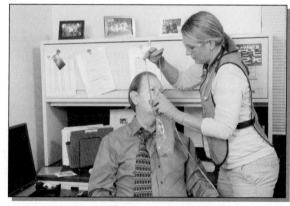

A2.3.4 Place the mask over the person's face, starting at the bridge of the nose and walking the mask down the face.

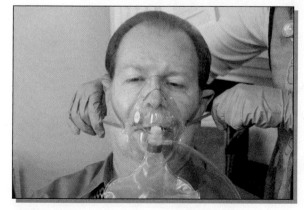

A2.3.5 Place the elastic band around the person's head, and pull the ends through the mask to ensure a snug fit.

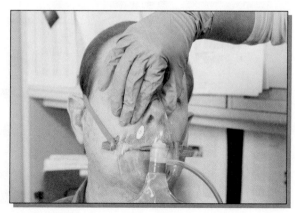

A2.3.6 Squeeze the aluminum nose strap to help seal the mask across the nose.

reservoir, it will deliver approximately 50 percent oxygen. Used with a reservoir, it will deliver nearly 100 percent oxygen.

Maintain an open airway and a tight mask-to-face seal, squeeze the bag to deliver oxygen, and release the bag to allow for a passive expiration. There is no need to remove the mask when the person exhales. This device also can be used to assist the breathing efforts of a person who has a slow respiratory rate (fewer than 10 breaths per minute). This device works best when used by two rescuers. The first rescuer obtains a tight mask-to-face seal and keeps the airway open. The second rescuer squeezes the bag with both hands.

Monitor the person carefully whenever you are providing assisted ventilations. High pressure caused by forcing air or oxygen into a person's airway can force air into the esophagus and fill the stomach. Air distends the stomach, which presses into the lung cavity and reduces expansion of the lungs. To avoid or correct this problem, carefully maintain and monitor airway, mask-to-face seal, and chest rise.

Using a Bag-Mask Device

For the best possible results, the bag mask should be used with two rescuers. One rescuer can use two hands to maintain a good mask seal, while the second rescuer squeezes the bag. Note also that for injured people who must have their airway opened by the jaw-thrust maneuver, the two-rescuer method is more effective. The rescuer holding the mask in place can more easily perform the jaw-thrust while the other rescuer provides effective rescue breaths.

Perform the following steps to provide rescue breaths using the two-rescuer bag-mask technique (Scan A2.4):

1. Take the appropriate BSI precautions.
2. Ensure an open airway, and position yourself at the person's head. Clear the airway if necessary.
3. Insert an airway adjunct if available.

MAKE A NOTE

A bag-mask device is not recommended when performing one-rescuer CPR. The preferred device for one-rescuer CPR is a pocket mask. ●

MAKE A NOTE

In some instances as a single rescuer, it may be more effective to provide assisted ventilations using the mouth-to-mask technique than attempting to use a bag-mask device by yourself. ●

SCAN A2.4   **Use of a Bag-Mask Device**

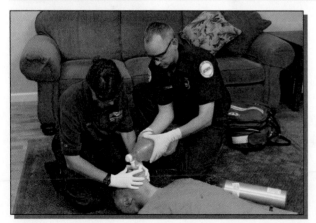

A2.4.1 Proper technique for using the bag-mask device with two responders.

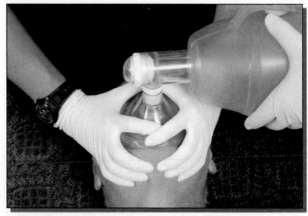

A2.4.2 Proper hand position for bag-mask ventilation with two responders.

4. Rescuer 1 should kneel at the top of the person's head, holding the mask firmly in place with both hands.

5. Rescuer 2 should kneel beside the person's head and connect the bag to the mask (if not already done). He should then squeeze the bag once every five to six seconds. Ensure adequate rise and fall of the chest each time the bag is squeezed.

Though not recommended, the bag-mask device also can be used during two-rescuer CPR by a single skilled operator. The rescuer providing ventilations uses two hands to maintain a face-mask seal and an open airway. The rescuer performing compressions, after providing 30 compressions, reaches over and squeezes the bag to provide two rescue breaths. They then resume chest compressions.

USE OF AN AIRWAY ADJUNCT

The use of a basic **airway adjunct** can assist the Emergency Responder in managing an ill or injured person's airway. The most common type of basic airway adjunct is the oropharyngeal airway (OPA). As you learn to use this device, it is very important to keep in mind that it is only an adjunct or aid to *assist* in managing a person's airway and breathing status. The OPA only helps the Emergency Responder maintain an open airway, allowing for more effective respirations or rescue breaths.

One disadvantage of all adjunct equipment is that it can delay the beginning of resuscitation if it is not readily available. Your pocket facemask and airway adjunct should always be handy. Never delay the start of rescue breaths or CPR while you try to find, retrieve, or set up airway adjunct equipment.

airway adjunct a device designed to assist in keeping an open and clear airway.

Oropharyngeal Airways

The prefix "oro" refers to the mouth. "Pharyngeo" refers to the throat. An oropharyngeal airway (OPA) is a device, usually made of rigid plastic, that can be inserted into a person's mouth. It has a flange that rests against the person's lips. The lower portion curves back into the throat and rests against the tongue, restricting its movement and minimizing the chance that it will block the airway. Once the airway is opened manually by using the head-tilt/chin-lift or jaw-thrust maneuver, an OPA may be inserted to help keep it open.

A2.7 Explain the indications and contraindication for the insertion of an oropharyngeal airway.

OPAs should only be used in unresponsive people who do not have a gag reflex. These devices can stimulate a person's normal gag reflex, causing him to vomit. If the unresponsive person vomits, he can aspirate, or breathe, the vomit back into his airway and lungs, causing a blockage and possibly a serious infection. If the person is responsive, even if disoriented or confused, or unresponsive with a gag reflex, do not insert an OPA. Do not continue to insert or leave the device in the person's mouth if you meet any resistance or if the person begins to gag as you insert it.

You already may see that the rules for deciding whether to use an OPA can be something of a contradiction. You are not supposed to use an OPA on a person with a gag reflex, yet you will not know if the person has one unless you attempt to insert the OPA first. To resolve this dilemma, you must be very focused as you insert the OPA. Expect that he may have a gag reflex, and at the first indication that he does, remove the airway.

If you carry a suction unit and are trained to use it, have it ready for any person who is unresponsive and may need an airway. You do not want to be caught unprepared when the person vomits.

Measuring the Oropharyngeal Airway

There are numerous sizes of OPAs designed to fit infants, children, and adults. To use this device effectively, you must be able to select the correct size for the person. Before inserting an airway, hold the device against the person's face to see if it extends from the center of the mouth to the angle of the lower jaw. If it does, it is the correct size. The airway also may be sized by holding it at the corner of the person's mouth and seeing if it will extend to the tip of the earlobe on the same side of the face.

Use an OPA only if it is the correct size. If it is not, select another airway and measure it to ensure it is the correct size before inserting.

An airway that is the wrong size has the potential to cause more harm than good. If the airway is too long, it might extend too far into the throat and block the airway. If the device is too short, it will not restrict the movement of the tongue, allowing it to block the airway.

Inserting the Oropharyngeal Airway

To insert an OPA, you should (Scan A2.5):

1. Take the appropriate BSI precautions.
2. With the person on his back (prone), manually open the airway using the head-tilt/chin-lift or jaw-thrust maneuver.
3. Select the appropriate-size airway by measuring from the middle of the mouth to the angle of the jaw or from the corner of the mouth to the earlobe.
4. Insert the airway by positioning it so that its tip is pointing toward the roof of the person's mouth.
5. Insert the airway and slide it along the roof of the mouth, being certain not to push the tongue back into the throat.
6. Once the airway is about halfway in, rotate it 180 degrees so that the tip is positioned at the base of the tongue. Allow the flange to rest against the outside of the lips.
7. Monitor the airway constantly. Check to see that the flange of the airway is against the person's lips. If the airway is too long, it will keep slipping out of the mouth and the flange will not rest on the lips. If the airway is too short, the person's mouth may remain slightly open in an awkward position.
8. Provide rescue breaths with the most appropriate technique.
9. Continue to monitor the person's airway closely. If the person becomes responsive, he may attempt to remove, displace, or cough up the airway. You must be ready to assist or remove it for him.

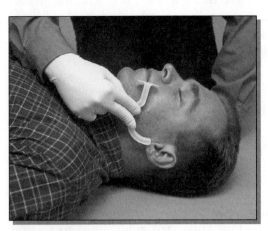

A2.5.1 Measure from the corner of the mouth to the tip of the earlobe.

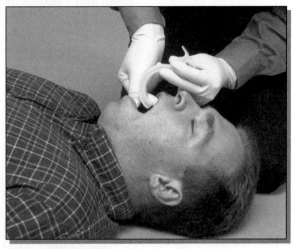

A2.5.2 Insert the airway with the tip pointing to the roof of the mouth.

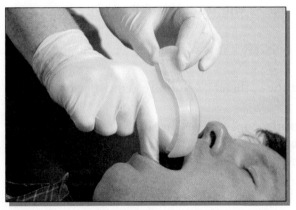

A2.5.3 An alternative method is to insert the airway sideways.

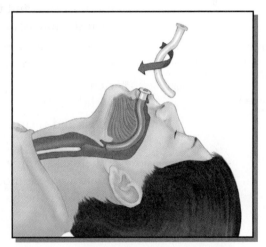

A2.5.4 Rotate the airway into position. When it is in place, the flange rests on the mouth.

An alternative method for inserting an OPA is to insert it sideways into the mouth until it is approximately halfway in. Then simply rotate it 90 degrees. Just as with the first method, make certain that the tip of the airway is positioned at the base of the tongue. This method is less likely to cause trauma to the roof of the person's mouth during insertion. As with all these skills, follow your instructor's preference as well as local protocols.

USING SUCTION

To clear blood, mucus, and other body fluids from a person's airway, an Emergency Responder will usually position the person on his side (recovery position) or use finger sweeps appropriately. However, a suction device can

A2.8 Explain the indications for oral suctioning.

assist in keeping a person's airway clear. There are several types of portable suction units available, including manually powered, oxygen- or air-powered, and electrically powered units.

All types of suction units must have thick-walled, non-kinking, wide-bore tubing; a nonbreakable collection container (bottle); and sterile, disposable, semirigid but flexible or rigid suction tips. The longer, flexible suction tips are usually called catheters. Rigid suction tips are sometimes referred to as tonsil suction tips.

General Guidelines for Suctioning

- Always use appropriate BSI precautions, including a mouth and eye shield since the potential for being sprayed with body fluids such as vomit, blood, and saliva is high.

- Keep your suctioning time to a minimum. Remember that while you are suctioning, you are not ventilating. Also, suction removes valuable oxygen along with dangerous fluids. One suggested guideline is to suction for no more than 15 seconds.

- If there is lots of fluid in the person's airway, it may be helpful to roll him onto his side and then suction. You may need to suction, ventilate, and then suction again in a continuous sequence as long as necessary.

suction catheter a device connected at the end of suction tubing that is used to suction fluids from a person's mouth and/or nose.

- Measure the **suction catheter** as you would an OPA before inserting it into the person's mouth.

- Activate the suction unit only after it is completely inserted and as you withdraw the catheter.

- Twist and turn the tip of the catheter as you are removing it from the mouth or nose.

- When suctioning the mouth, concentrate on the back corners of the mouth, where most fluids tend to accumulate. Do not place the tip directly over the back of the tongue, because this will likely stimulate the gag reflex.

Suctioning Technique

There are many variations to the techniques used to suction the mouth or nose. You should follow your own local protocols for how to suction a person who needs it, but general guidelines are as follows (Scan A2.6):

1. Before suctioning, be sure to take the appropriate BSI precautions.
2. Attach the catheter and activate the unit to ensure that there is suction.
3. Position yourself at the person's head. If possible, turn the person onto his side. Follow guidelines for protection of the spine.
4. Measure the catheter prior to insertion.
5. Open the person's mouth and clear obvious matter and fluid from the oral cavity by letting the mouth drain or by using finger sweeps with a gloved hand.

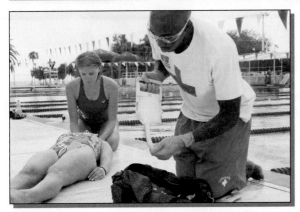

A2.6.1 Attach the catheter and activate the unit to ensure that there is suction.

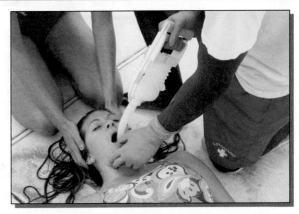

A2.6.2 Open the person's mouth and insert the tip of the catheter to the appropriate depth.

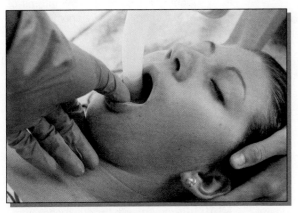

A2.6.3 Suction one side and then the other. Remain alert for signs of a gag reflex and vomiting.

6. Insert the tip of the catheter to the appropriate depth. Usually, the tip is inserted to the base of the tongue. If you are using a rigid catheter, place the convex (curved-out) side against the roof of the mouth with the tip at the base of the tongue.

7. Apply suction only when the tip or catheter is in place at the back of the mouth or base of the tongue and as you begin to withdraw it. Twist and turn it from side to side and sweep the mouth. This twisting action prevents the end of the catheter from grabbing the soft tissue inside the mouth.

8. Remain alert for signs of a gag reflex and vomiting.

Appendix 3

Weapons of Mass Destruction and the Terrorist Threat

LEARNING OBJECTIVES

At the conclusion of this appendix and the associated instructor-guided lesson, the student will be able to:

Cognitive

A3.1 List the five most common types of weapons of mass destruction. *(p. 209)*

A3.2 List the three types of radioactive particles. *(p. 209)*

A3.3 List the four types of biological agents. *(p. 210)*

A3.4 List the five classifications of chemical agents. *(p. 210)*

A3.5 Recognize the warning signs of a chemical nerve agent/mass exposure incident. *(p. 210)*

A3.6 Identify the signs and symptoms of exposure to a chemical nerve agent product. *(p. 210)*

A3.7 Explain the emergency treatment for a chemical nerve agent. *(p. 210)*

A3.8 Recognize the warning signs of a chemical nerve agent/mass exposure incident. *(p. 211)*

A3.9 Identify the signs and symptoms of exposure to a chemical nerve agent product. *(p. 211)*

A3.10 Be familiar with the emergency treatment for a chemical nerve agent. *(p. 211)*

Introduction

terrorism the unlawful use of force and violence against persons or property to intimidate or coerce a government, the civilian population, or any segment thereof to further political or any segment thereof, in furtherance of political or social objectives.

THE U.S. government defines **terrorism** as "the unlawful use of force and violence against persons or property to intimidate or coerce a government, the civilian population, or any segment thereof to further political or any segment thereof, in furtherance of political or social objectives."[1] For years, the people of the United States remained somewhat insulated from the effects of terrorists and terrorism, since they only viewed such events on the nightly news. However, terrorism is no longer something that only happens in distant countries.

---

[1]Federal Bureau of Investigation, *FBI Publication #0308: Terrorism 2000/2001: FBI Policy and Guidelines.* (Washington, DC: U.S. Department of Justice, n.d.), http://www.fbi.gov/publications/terror/terror2000_2001. htm (accessed January 1, 2010).

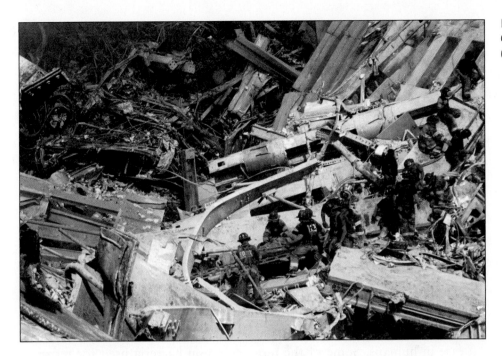

Figure A3.1 World Trade Center, September 2001 (© David Turnley/Corbis)

In recent years, the effects of terrorism have hit home with incidents such as the bombing of the Federal Building in Oklahoma City, the spread of anthrax through the U.S. Postal Service, and the events of September 11, 2001, in New York (▲ Figure A3.1), Washington DC, and rural Pennsylvania.

INCIDENTS INVOLVING NUCLEAR/ RADIOLOGICAL AGENTS

Until recently, the potential for a terrorist organization to obtain or develop nuclear devices was thought to be minimal. With the growing supply of nuclear waste on a worldwide scale and the developing technology of third-world countries, the likelihood of a nuclear threat by a terrorist organization is ever increasing.

There are two types of potential nuclear incidents. One is the possible detonation of a nuclear device, and the other is the detonation of a conventional explosive that incorporates nuclear material. A plausible scenario involves the detonation of a **radiological dispersal device (RDD)**, which would spread radioactive material for a wide area surrounding the blast site. Another scenario involves the detonation of a large explosive device (such as a truck bomb) near a nuclear power plant or radiological cargo transport.

Nuclear incidents emit three main types of radioactive particles:

- **Alpha particles.** These are the heaviest and most highly charged of the nuclear particles. They are easily stopped by human skin but can become a serious hazard if ingested or inhaled.

- **Beta particles.** Smaller and able to travel much faster and farther than alpha particles, beta particles can penetrate the skin but rarely reach the vital organs. While they can cause burns to the skin if exposure lasts long

A3.1 List the five most common types of weapons of mass destruction.

radiological dispersal device (RDD) a device that can spread radioactive material for a wide area surrounding a blast site.

A3.2 List the three types of radioactive particles.

enough, the biggest threat occurs when they are ingested or inhaled into the body. Beta particles also can enter the body through unprotected open wounds.

- **Gamma rays.** These are a type of radiation that travels through the air in the form of waves. The rays can travel great distances and penetrate most materials, including the human body. Acute radiation sickness occurs when someone is exposed to large doses of gamma radiation over a short period of time and can cause symptoms such as skin irritation, burns, nausea, vomiting, high fever, and hair loss.

INCIDENTS INVOLVING BIOLOGICAL AGENTS

A3.3 List the four types of biological agents.

Biological agents pose one of the most serious threats due to their accessibility and ability to spread rapidly. The potential is also very high for widespread casualties. Biological agents are most dangerous when either inhaled (spread through the air) or ingested (through contaminated food or water supplies).

There are four common types of biological agents:

- **Bacteria.** These are single-celled organisms that can quickly cause disease in humans. Some of the more common bacteria used for terrorist activities are anthrax, cholera, the plague, and tularemia.
- **Rickettsia.** Smaller than bacteria cells, rickettsia live inside individual host cells. An example of rickettsia is *Coxiella burnetii*, which is the organism that causes Q fever.
- **Viruses.** The simplest of microorganisms, viruses cannot survive without a living host. The most common viruses that have served as biological agents include smallpox, Venezuelan equine encephalitis, and Ebola, among others.
- **Toxins.** These are substances that occur naturally in the environment and can be produced by an animal, plant, or microbe. They differ from biological agents in that they are not manufactured. The four common toxins with a history of use as terrorist weapons are botulism, SEB (staphylococcal enterotoxin), ricin, and mycotoxins. Ricin has been used in several well-publicized incidents in the United States and Japan. It is a toxin made from the castor bean plant, which is grown all over the world.

INCIDENTS INVOLVING CHEMICAL AGENTS

A3.4 List the five classifications of chemical agents.

A3.5 Recognize the warning signs of a chemical nerve agent/mass exposure incident.

A3.6 Identify the signs and symptoms of exposure to a chemical nerve agent product.

A3.7 Explain the emergency treatment for a chemical nerve agent.

The primary routes of exposure for chemical agents are inhalation, ingestion, and absorption, or contact with the skin—with inhalation being the most common. The five classifications of chemical agents are nerve agents, vesicant (blister) agents, cyanogens agents, pulmonary agents, and riot-control agents.

Nerve Agents

Nerve agents are highly poisonous chemicals and the most toxic of the known chemical warfare agents. They disrupt nerve impulse transmissions throughout the body and are extremely toxic in very small quantities. They poison the nervous system of those who are exposed, affecting movement and breathing.[2] In some cases, a single small drop can be fatal to the average human being.

Nerve agents have been used by terrorists and pose a real threat to Emergency Responders. Nerve agents include sarin (GB), soman (GD), tabun (GA), and V agent (VX). These are liquid agents that have been used against Japanese and Iraqi civilians and are typically spread in the form of an aerosol spray

In the case of GA, GB, and GD, the G stands for the country (Germany) that developed the agent. The second letter indicates the order in which the agent was developed. In the case of VX, the V stands for venom and the X represents one of the chemicals that make up the compound. These agents resemble water or clear oil in their purest form and possess no odor. Sometimes small explosives are used to spread them, which can cause widespread death. Many dead animals at the scene of an incident may be a warning sign or clue.

Early signs of nerve agent exposure are:

- Uncontrolled salivation.
- Urination.
- Defecation.
- Tearing.

Other later signs and symptoms include:

- Blurred vision.
- Excessive sweating.
- Muscle tremors.
- Difficulty breathing.
- Nausea, vomiting.
- Abdominal pain.

A3.8 Recognize the warning signs of a chemical nerve agent/mass exposure incident.

A3.9 Identify the signs and symptoms of exposure to a chemical nerve agent product.

Emergency treatment for nerve agent exposure includes the use of medications that counteract the agent's effects. Nerve agent autoinjectors (e.g., DuoDote) contain two medications—atropine and pralidoxime chloride—that counteract the effects of exposure. To achieve maximum effectiveness, these antidotes must be administered as quickly as possible by EMS personnel who have had adequate training in the recognition and treatment of chemical nerve agents. Nerve agent autoinjectors are FDA approved for use by EMS personnel and available only with a prescription.[3] The autoinjection site is the mid-outer thigh area and can inject through clothing (pockets at the injection site must be empty).

A3.10 Be familiar with the emergency treatment for a chemical nerve agent.

Vesicant Agents

Vesicant agents are more commonly referred to as blister or mustard agents due to their unique smell. They can easily penetrate several layers of clothing

---

[2]Centers for Disease Control and Prevention, Emergency Preparedness and Response: Nerve Agents (Atlanta: Centers for Disease Control and Prevention, n.d.), http://www.bt.cdc.gov/agent/nerve/ (accessed January 1, 2010).

[3]Meridian Medical Technologies, Inc., "Prescribing Information" [package insert] (Columbia, MD: Meridian Medical Technologies, n.d.), http://www.meridianmeds.com/pdf/DuoDote_Pack_Insert.pdf (accessed January 1, 2010).

and are quickly absorbed into the skin. Mustard (H, HD, HN) and Lewisite (L, HL) are common vesicants. Although less toxic than nerve agents, it takes only a few drops on the skin to cause severe injury.

The signs and symptoms of vesicant exposure include:

- Reddening, swelling, and tearing of the eyes.
- Tenderness and burning of the skin followed by the development of fluid-filled blisters.
- Nausea, vomiting.
- Severe abdominal pain.
- Runny nose, burning in the throat, and shortness of breath about two hours post exposure

Cyanogens

Cyanogens are agents that interfere with the ability of the blood to carry oxygen and can cause asphyxiation in victims of exposure. Common cyanogens are hydrogen cyanide (AC) and cyanogen chloride (CK). All cyanogens are very toxic in high concentrations and can lead to rapid death. Under pressure, these agents are in liquid form. In their pure form, they are a gas. Cyanogens are common industrial chemicals used in a variety of processes, and all have an aroma similar to bitter almonds or peach blossoms.

Signs and symptoms of cyanogens exposure include:

- Severe respiratory distress.
- Vomiting.
- Diarrhea.
- Dizziness, headache.
- Seizures, coma.

It is essential that victims of exposure be moved quickly to fresh air and treated for respiratory distress.

Pulmonary Agents

Pulmonary agents are sometimes called *choking agents*. They directly affect the respiratory system, causing fluid buildup (edema) in the lungs, which in turn causes asphyxiation similar to that seen in drowning victims. Chlorine and phosgene are two of the most common of these agents and are usually found in industrial settings. Chlorine is a familiar smell to most people. Phosgene has an aroma of freshly cut hay. Both of these chemicals are in a gaseous state in their pure form and are stored in bottles or cylinders. Signs and symptoms include:

- Severe eye irritation.
- Coughing.
- Choking.
- Severe respiratory distress.

Riot-Control Agents

Riot-control agents include both irritating and psychedelic agents, both of which are designed to incapacitate the victim. For the most part, they are not lethal, but under certain circumstances irritating agents have been known to cause asphyxiation. In some individuals, psychedelic agents have been known to cause behavior that can lead to death.

Common irritating agents include mace, tear gas, and pepper spray. These agents typically cause severe pain when they come in contact with the skin, especially moist areas such as the nose, mouth, and eyes.

Signs and symptoms of exposure to irritating agents include:

- Burning and irritation in the eyes and throat.
- Coughing, choking.
- Respiratory distress.
- Nausea.
- Vomiting.

Psychedelic agents include lysergic acid diethylamide (LSD), 3-quinuclidinyl benzilate (BZ), and benactyzine. These agents alter the nervous system causing visual and aural hallucinations and severe changes in thought processes and behavior. The effects of these agents can be unpredictable, ranging from overwhelming fear to extreme belligerence.

ROLE OF THE EMERGENCY RESPONDER

Terrorist attacks are meant to cause fear, and they are likely to occur when they are least expected. Having a high index of suspicion and recognizing the outward warning signs of a possible terrorist attack is of utmost importance for Emergency Responders. The primary protection against exposure to chemical nerve agents is donning the appropriate personal protective equipment, including masks designed specifically for this use.

Firefighters are probably the best prepared of all Emergency Responders because of the wide range of duties they are trained and expected to perform. Most other types of Emergency Responders are probably less equipped to respond to a terrorist attack because their personal protective equipment is primarily designed to minimize exposure to body fluids.

Without the proper training and equipment, Emergency Responders are likely to become victims if they enter the scene too quickly. In most cases, the best action will be to recognize the danger as soon as possible and retreat to a safe distance from the scene. Requesting appropriate resources such as specialized hazardous-materials teams will be important.

Note: Many terrorists will set a secondary device that is meant to incapacitate or kill responders. These devices may be set to go off 10 to 15 minutes after the first one. By doing this, terrorists will be sure that the device will go off while rescuers are caring for persons who were injured by the first one. Make sure that the scene is truly safe before entering.

DECONTAMINATION

decontamination removal of harmful substances such as noxious chemicals, harmful bacteria or other organisms, or radioactive material from exposed individuals.

Decontamination is the process by which chemical, biological, and/or radiological agents are removed from exposed victims, equipment, and the environment. Regardless if the incident is a hazardous-materials release or an intentional terrorist act, prompt decontamination can be the single most important aspect of the operation to minimize exposure and limit casualties. *If you have been exposed to a nerve agent, remove all clothing immediately and wash with copious amounts of soap and water. Seek immediate emergency medical attention.*

Depending on the size and scope of the incident, Emergency Responders may be asked to assist with the decontamination process. If not a part of the decontamination process, they will certainly play an important role in the emergency care given to ill or injured persons after they have gone through decontamination. It will be important for Emergency Responders assisting at such an event to continue to wear the appropriate personal protective equipment even after a victim has been decontaminated. This will minimize any contamination from residual agents remaining on the victim or equipment. *Emergency Responders assisting evacuated victims of nerve agent poisoning must avoid contaminating themselves by exposure to the victim's clothing.*

Appendix 4

Skill Sheets

This appendix contains five skill sheets that are designed to help you learn and practice the specific steps for each individual skill. You can use these by yourself to begin memorizing the steps necessary for each skill, or you can use them to test one another as you practice skills with your fellow students.

It is important to understand that skill sheets are very linear in nature and do not always accurately reflect how care should be provided when there is more than one care provider. Practicing with these skill sheets will help reinforce the priority of each step and the general order in which each step should be performed. In many cases, during a real emergency, some care steps can and should be performed simultaneously when more than one care provider is available.

Airway Management

Steps to be Performed	Action/Verbal Response	Completed
*Takes or verbalizes appropriate body substance isolation (BSI) precautions	I will take appropriate BSI precautions.	
Opening the Airway		
Performs appropriate method for opening the airway	I will perform a head-tilt/chin-lift or jaw-thrust maneuver, depending on the mechanism of injury.	
Assesses for breathing status	I will place my ear next to the person's nose and mouth and assess for breathing for 5 to 10 seconds.	
The Examiner states: The person appears to be breathing adequately but is unresponsive.		
Repositions person and monitors breathing status	I will position the person based on the mechanism of injury and closely monitor ABCs until EMS arrives.	

(Optional)

Oropharyngeal Airway (OPA)		
Selects appropriate airway	I will select the appropriate airway and the approximate size.	
Measures airway	I will measure the airway from the corner of the mouth to the earlobe.	
Inserts airway	I will insert the airway in a manner that will not push the tongue back into the patient's airway.	
The Examiner states: The patient is gagging and becoming responsive.		
Properly removes airway	I will remove the airway by pulling it straight out.	

Date: _____

Student's Name: _____

Evaluator's Name: _____

Bleeding Control/Shock Management

Steps to be Performed	Action/Verbal Response	Completed
*Takes or states appropriate body substance isolation (BSI) precautions	I will take appropriate BSI precautions.	
*Applies direct pressure to wound	Using an appropriate dressing, I am applying direct pressure to the wound.	
The Examiner states: The wound continues to bleed.		
*Applies a tourniquet	I will apply a tourniquet just proximal to the wound and tighten until the bleeding stops.	
The Examiner states: The bleeding is now controlled. The patient is showing signs and symptoms of shock (hypoperfusion).		
Properly positions the patient	I will lie the patient flat (supine).	
Initiates appropriate oxygen therapy (Optional)	I will place the patient on supplemental oxygen.	
Initiates steps to prevent heat loss from the patient	I will cover the patient with a blanket to preserve heat.	
*Indicates need for immediate transportation	I will categorize this patient as high priority for transport.	

*Critical criteria

Date: _____

Student's Name: _____

Evaluator's Name: _____

Immobilization: Joint Injury

Steps to be Performed	Action/Verbal Response	Completed
*Takes or states appropriate body substance isolation (BSI) precautions	I will take appropriate BSI precautions.	
Directs assistant/patient to initiate/maintain manual stabilization of the injury	I will direct my partner or the patient to manually stabilize the injury.	
*Assesses distal circulation, sensation, and motor function (CSM) in the injured extremity	I will assess the status of circulation, sensation, and motor function in the injured extremity.	
The Examiner states: Distal CSM is within normal limits.		
Selects proper splinting materials	I will select the appropriate materials/device that I will use to immobilize the extremity.	
*Immobilizes the injury site	I will apply the appropriate material/device to immobilize the injury site.	
*Immobilizes bone/joint above the injury site	I will apply the appropriate material/device to immobilize the bone/joint above the injury site.	
*Immobilizes bone/joint below the injury site	I will apply the appropriate material/device to immobilize the bone/joint below the injury site.	
*Reassesses distal circulation, sensation, and motor function in the injured extremity	I will reassess the status of circulation, sensation, and motor function in the injured extremity.	
The Examiner states: Distal CSM is within normal limits.		

*Critical criteria

Date: _____

Student's Name: _____

Evaluator's Name: _____

Immobilization: Long Bone

Steps to be Performed	Action/Verbal Response	Completed
*Takes or states appropriate body substance isolation (BSI) precautions	I will take appropriate BSI precautions.	
Directly applies manual stabilization to injury site	I will either direct the patient to continue holding the injury or ask my partner to take over for the patient.	
*Assesses circulation, sensation, and motor (DSM) function	I will now assess circulation, sensation, and motor function of the extremity.	
The Examiner states: Distal DSM is present and normal.		
Measures immobilization device	I will select an appropriate device and size it to ensure that it will fit the extremity.	
Applies device	I will apply the device to the extremity, ensuring that it is well padded.	
*Immobilizes joint above the injury site	I will immobilize the joint above the injury site.	
*Immobilizes the joint below the injury site	I will immobilize the joint below the injury site.	
Secures entire extremity	I will secure the entire extremity to minimize movement.	
Ensures hand/foot in position of function	I will ensure that the hand/foot is in the position of function.	

*Critical criteria

Date: _____

Student's Name: _____

Evaluator's Name: _____

Patient Assessment: Trauma

Determine Proper BSI	Action/Verbal Response	Completed
*Takes or verbalizes appropriate body substance isolation (BSI) precautions	I will take appropriate BSI precautions.	

Scene Size Up	Action/Verbal Response	
*Assesses scene safety	I will determine if the scene is safe.	
Determines mechanism of injury	I will determine the mechanism of injury.	
Determines number of patients	I will determine the number of patients.	
Assesses need for additional help	I will determine the need for additional help.	
Takes cervical spine precautions as necessary	I will take/direct appropriate c-spine precautions.	

Initial Assessment	Action/Verbal Response	
Determines responsiveness/ level of consciousness	**EYES OPEN/AWAKE:** "Hello, my name is _____. May I help you? What is your name? How old are you?" I have determined that the patient is awake and alert. **EYES CLOSED:** Determine responsiveness using: **A**lert - **V**erbal - **P**ainful - **U**nresponsive	
Determines chief complaint/ identifies apparent life threats	"What seems to be the problem?" I will identify and address any obvious life threats.	
*Assesses airway/initiates appropriate airway management	**IF PATIENT SPEAKS TO YOU:** I have determined that the airway is open. **IF PATIENT DOES NOT SPEAK OR IS UNCONSCIOUS:** I am assessing for a clear and open airway.	
*Assess breathing/initiate appropriate oxygen therapy	I am assessing breathing for adequate rate and tidal volume, labored or easy. At this time, I would initiate oxygen therapy if appropriate. (Specify the device and appropriate flow rate.)	

(continued)

(continued)

*Assesses circulation	I am assessing for presence of a pulse at the carotid artery (unresponsive) or radial artery (responsive), assessing approximate rate, strength, and rhythm.	
*Assesses and controls severe bleeding	I am assessing for and controlling severe bleeding.	
Assesses skin signs	I am assessing the skin for color, temperature, and moisture.	
OBTAIN BASELINE VITAL SIGNS	I will obtain a baseline blood pressure, pulse, and respirations. Skin signs have already been noted. Pupils will be noted in secondary assessment.	**(1)**

Obtain **SAMPLE** history if patient is responsive.		
*S – Signs and symptoms of present injury	I will observe for obvious trauma and question the patient about his complaints: "Tell me again where you have pain."	
*A – Allergies	"Do you have any allergies to foods or medications?"	
*M – Medications	"Do you take any medications?" (prescribed/non-prescribed, vitamins, herbal remedies, birth control pills, recreational drugs)	
*P – Past pertinent medical history	"Has this ever happened before? When was the last time you saw a physician? Diagnosis? Do you have a history of diabetes, high blood pressure, cardiac or breathing problems, or seizures?"	
*L – Last oral intake	"What and when did you last eat or drink?"	
*E – Event(s) leading to present injury	"What happened today that led you or someone else to call for help?"	

(continued)

(continued)

Secondary Assessment		
Place an X in the box if the student performs an appropriate physical exam while stating the appropriate findings.	**B**leeding, **P**ain, **D**eformities, **O**pen wounds, **C**repitus	
Head	**I will examine the head for BPDOC.**	
Face	**I will examine the face for BPDOC** + *equality of facial muscles.*	
Eyes	**I will examine the eyes for size, equality, reactivity to light.**	
Ears	**I will examine the ears for BPDOC, drainage.**	
Nose	**I will examine the nose for BPDOC, drainage.**	
Mouth	**I will examine the mouth for BPDOC, loose/broken teeth, foreign body.**	
Neck	**I will examine the neck for BPDOC,** *medical identification jewelry.*	
Chest	**I will examine the chest for BPDOC, equal chest rise.**	
Abdomen	**I will examine the abdomen for BPDOC.**	
Pelvis	**I will examine the pelvis for BPDOC** + *incontinence.*	
Legs	**I will examine the legs for BPDOC, distal CSM,** *medical identification jewelry.*	
Arms	**I will examine the arms for distal BPDOC, distal CSM,** *medical identification jewelry.*	
Back	**I will examine the back for BPDOC.**	

Ongoing Assessment *(verbalized)*		
Obtains second set of vital signs and compares to baseline	I will record a second set of vital signs and compare with the first set.	
*= Critical criteria		

Student's Name: _____

Evaluator's Name: _____

Answers

CHAPTER 1

Quick Check

Question: What is the highest level of EMS training for the individual who can be found on ambulances and fire engines and in helicopters across the nation?
Answer: Paramedic.

Question: Which is the most efficient way to contact local resources in the event of an emergency—using a landline or a cell phone to call 911?
Answer: A land line.

Quick Quiz

1. b
2. c
3. c
4. d
5. b

CHAPTER 2

Quick Check

Question: When is it necessary for you to remain at the emergency scene or with the injured or ill person?
Answer: By stopping and assisting an ill or injured person, you have legally established duty and must remain with the person until someone of equal or higher training takes over for you.

Quick Quiz

1. b
2. c
3. d
4. a
5. b

CHAPTER 3

Quick Check

Question: Is it ever appropriate to help another person if it puts you at an unreasonable risk?
Answer: No. Responding without concern for personal safety is reckless and unacceptable.

Question: Standard precautions are meant to protect you from exposure to potentially infectious blood and bodily fluids from which types of ill or injured people?
Answer: The underlying philosophy is that *all* ill or injured people (universally) should be considered potentially infectious and that you should take the necessary precautions to properly minimize exposure to body fluids.

Quick Quiz

1. d
2. a
3. b
4. c
5. a
6. b
7. d

CHAPTER 4

Quick Check

Question: Describe a person who is in the anatomical position.
Answer: A person in the anatomical position is standing upright with arms extended down at the sides and the palms of the hands facing forward.

Question: Which of the four main body cavities can hide enough blood loss to be life threatening?
Answer: Chest, abdomen, pelvis.

Question: Blood traveling from the right side of the heart goes where?
Answer: Blood traveling from the right side of the heart goes to the lungs, where it receives oxygen before returning to the left side of the heart.

Quick Quiz

1. c
2. c
3. a
4. b
5. d
6. c
7. b

CHAPTER 5

Quick Check

Question: Which is the best way to avoid injury—holding a heavy object close or far from your body?
Answer: Keep the weight as close to your body as possible. Keeping the weight close keeps it centered and minimizes strain on the back.

Question: For what ill or injured person is the extremity lift ideally suited?

Answer: Use an extremity lift when an ill or injured person, who does *not* have a suspected neck or back injury, must be lifted from the ground to a chair, couch, or some type of stretcher.

Quick Quiz

1. b
2. a
3. c
4. d
5. c

CHAPTER 6

Quick Check

Question: Which problem requires the most immediate response—a partial airway obstruction or a complete obstruction? Explain your reasoning.

Answer: A complete obstruction prevents any air from moving through the airway and must be corrected immediately. Partial obstructions still allow for some movement of air through the airway and are typically not as life threatening.

Question: For you to perform an adequate airway and breathing check of an ill or injured person who is unresponsive, what position must the ill or injured person be in?

Answer: To perform an adequate airway and breathing check of an ill or injured person who is unresponsive, the person must be in a supine (face-up) position.

Question: Should a head-tilt/chin-lift ever be attempted on a person with a suspected neck or back injury? Explain your answer.

Answer: If you are unable to adequately maintain an open airway using the jaw-thrust maneuver, you must move to the head-tilt/chin-lift maneuver, regardless of neck or back injury. An open and clear airway is more important than the risk of causing further injury to the neck or back.

Question: What are the signs and symptoms of respiratory difficulty?

Answer: Signs and symptoms of respiratory difficulty include increased breathing rate, increased work of breathing, panicked look, obvious movement of chest and abdomen, and use of neck muscles to breathe.

Quick Quiz

1. a
2. b
3. c
4. a
5. c
6. a

7. d
8. a
9. b
10. d

CHAPTER 7

Quick Check

Question: What is the term used to describe the general cause of a person's injury? Of a person's illness?
Answer: The term used to describe the general cause of a person's injury is "mechanism of injury." The term used to describe the general cause of a person's illness is "nature of illness."

Question: Should you perform a primary assessment before or after the scene size-up?
Answer: Perform a primary assessment of the ill or injured person only after you have performed a scene size-up and made sure that the scene is safe to enter.

Question: In what part of the SAMPLE history might you learn that the person you are caring for had a heart attack six months ago?
Answer: You are likely to learn that the person you are caring for had a heart attack six months ago while asking about his "pertinent medical history (P)."

Question: Is the assessment process different or the same for an unresponsive person compared to a responsive person? Explain your reasoning.
Answer: When caring for an unresponsive person, it is not possible to obtain any information from the person verbally. So you must rely on what you see during your physical examination and information gathered from bystanders.

Question: Why is documentation important to the process of caring for a person who is ill or injured?
Answer: Documentation helps to ensure that everyone who will be caring for a person knows what has already been done.

Quick Quiz

1. b
2. d
3. a
4. a
5. b
6. c
7. a
8. d
9. b
10. d

CHAPTER 8

Quick Check

Question: If there is a problem with the primary assessment, must you still do your best to complete a secondary assessment before EMS arrives? Why or why not?
Answer: No. The primary assessment deals with airway, breathing, circulation, and bleeding. If there is an issue with any of these, you must not move on until it has been properly addressed.

Question: Assuming that the scene is safe, what is your top priority when caring for a person who is actively convulsing from a seizure?
Answer: Your top priority should be to protect the person from further injury until the convulsions stop. Then your priority will be airway and breathing.

Question: What is the ideal position for anyone with an altered mental status who does not have a neck or back injury?
Answer: The recovery position. This will help maintain an open and clear airway.

Question: Is it appropriate to encourage a person to take his medication whether it has expired or not?
Answer: No. Medication should never be taken if it has expired.

Question: Heat stroke is a life-threatening condition. What is your priority of care?
Answer: The priority of care for heat stroke is to first ensure that the ABCs are okay. Once that is done, the next priority is to cool the person.

Quick Quiz

1. c
2. d
3. c
4. b
5. d
6. a
7. c
8. b
9. d
10. a

CHAPTER 9

Quick Check

Question: Bleeding from which type of vessel is the most difficult to control?
Answer: Bleeding from arteries is often the most difficult to control due to the higher pressure contained within these vessels.

Question: What is it called when the organs and cells of the body do not receive an adequate supply of well-oxygenated blood?

Answer: Shock is the condition that results when the cells of the body do not receive an adequate supply of well-oxygenated blood.

Question: What is the name of the material that is designed to be applied directly to a wound to assist with bleeding control?
Answer: A dressing is designed to be placed directly over a wound. It can be clean or sterile and should extend beyond the wound on all sides. A bandage secures a dressing to the wound.

Question: Your attempts to control bleeding with direct pressure and elevation have failed. What should be your next step?
Answer: If direct pressure and elevation fail to control the bleeding, the next step is to apply a tourniquet.

Question: How should an amputated part be handled by the Emergency Responder?
Answer: An amputated part should be wrapped in dry gauze and placed on ice until EMS personnel arrives.

Question: What is the most appropriate method for caring for closed burns?
Answer: Closed burns can be cared for by running cool water over the burns.

Quick Quiz

1. c
2. b
3. d
4. c
5. b
6. a
7. d
8. d
9. b
10. c
11. a
12. c

CHAPTER 10

Quick Check

Question: Which structure holds two or more bones together at a joint?
Answer: Ligaments are tough, fiber-like tissues that connect two or more bones, typically at a joint.

Question: Should bleeding from an open injury be controlled before or after the injured limb has been immobilized?
Answer: The control of blood loss is a higher priority than the immobilization of suspected fractures. A person can die from too much blood loss, but he will not die because you were delayed in splinting an injury. Always control the bleeding of an open injury before attempting to immobilize the injured limb.

Question: What are two signs of deformity in a musculoskeletal injury?
Answer: Both swelling and angulation can be signs of deformity when found in an extremity. These signs may be an indication of an underlying fracture or dislocation.

Question: What information about an extremity does capillary refill provide?
Answer: It helps to determine the status of circulation beyond the injury site. It is important to know that a cold environment and some medical conditions can cause poor capillary refill. When capillary refill seems poor or absent, always compare the injured side to the uninjured side.

Question: When is "self-splinting" an acceptable method of stabilizing or immobilizing an injured extremity?
Answer: If the situation will allow it, and EMS personnel is expected to arrive on scene in a short time, it may be appropriate to allow the injured person to self-splint and wait. Attempting to immobilize may cause too much pain and discomfort for the injured person.

Question: In addition to self-splinting, manual stabilization, and splinting, what additional emergency care can be performed that will help decrease bleeding, swelling, pain, and disability?
Answer: Apply cold to the injured area with a plastic bag or damp cloth filled with ice. To prevent cold injury, place a thin towel or cloth between the cold source and the skin, and limit application to 20 minutes or less.

Quick Quiz

1. a
2. b
3. d
4. c
5. a
6. b

CHAPTER 11

Quick Check

Question: Which part of the body is responsible for regulating many of the body's involuntary functions?
Answer: The central nervous system, which is made up of the brain and the spinal cord, is responsible for many of the body's involuntary functions.

Question: A person with a head injury should be cared for as if he has what other type of injury?
Answer: Any person with a head injury is at risk of also having a neck injury. You must provide manual stabilization of the head and neck until EMS arrives.

Question: Why is the jaw-thrust maneuver preferred for an injured person with a suspected neck injury?
Answer: When opening the airway of a person with a suspected neck injury, the jaw-thrust maneuver minimizes the movement of the neck and any chances of causing further harm to the patient. Remember that if you are

unable to establish an open airway using the jaw-thrust, then use the head-tilt/chin-lift maneuver.

Question: Which part of the spine is located in the neck and consists of seven vertebrae?
Answer: The cervical spine is located in the neck, and it consists of seven vertebrae.

Quick Quiz

1. d
2. c
3. b
4. b
5. d
6. c
7. c

CHAPTER 12

Quick Check

Question: What is the commonly accepted definition of the term *multiple-casualty incident*?
Answer: One of the most widely accepted definitions of an MCI is any incident involving two or more ill or injured people that overwhelms the normal Emergency Responders or resources.

Question: What responsibilities do you have as an Emergency Responder at the scene of an MCI?
Answer: Your initial responsibilities when faced with a possible MCI are to identify the emergency as a multiple-casualty incident, ensure your personal safety and that of any bystanders, give as much information as possible about the incident to the 911 dispatcher, and serve as a resource for EMS personnel.

Question: According to a basic triage system, which of the ill or injured would be categorized as deceased?
Answer: People who have no signs of life and would require multiple resources to attempt resuscitation are categorized initially as deceased. If adequate resources arrive on the scene, it is not unheard of to re-triage these people and initiate additional care as appropriate.

Quick Quiz

1. a
2. d
3. c
4. b
5. d
6. a
7. b

CHAPTER 13

Quick Check

Question: Where does the fertilized egg attach itself to grow and develop for 40 weeks?
Answer: After the egg is fertilized, it implants on the inside wall of the uterus, where it will spend the next 40 weeks developing into a full-size baby.

Question: What is labor, and how is it characterized?
Answer: Labor is the process the woman's body goes through to deliver a fetus. It is characterized by gradually increasing contractions of the muscular uterus as it works to push the baby out during delivery.

Question: What is the best way to determine the interval between contractions?
Answer: One of the indications of how soon the birth will occur is the time between contractions, or contraction interval. The shorter the interval, the more likely birth will occur. To determine how far apart contractions are, you must note the time at the beginning of a contraction and then count the time until the beginning of the next one.

Question: What are some indications that a delivery is imminent?
Answer: Signs that a delivery is imminent include a mother who is at or near her due date, contractions that are less than five minutes apart, and the presence of crowning. Another sign that birth is imminent is the mother feeling a sensation to bear down (move her bowels). This is often a sign that the baby has progressed out of the uterus and into the vagina.

Question: What is your first priority following the delivery of the baby's head?
Answer: The first priority following the delivery of the baby's head is to suction the nose and mouth to help clear the airway of fluids. This is usually accomplished by using a small bulb-type syringe that can be found in the typical OB kit.

Question: What is your course of action when a newborn infant is not breathing?
Answer: If attempts to stimulate the baby to breathe have failed, you must initiate CPR, beginning with chest compressions. Continue CPR until the baby begins crying or EMS personnel arrives and takes over.

Question: How does asking a mother to pant through a contraction help during a complicated delivery such as a prolapsed cord?
Answer: Asking a mother to pant during a contraction will help minimize her desire to hold her breath and push. This will help to delay the birth until EMS personnel arrives.

Quick Quiz

1. b
2. d
3. c
4. c
5. a
6. d
7. b
8. c

Glossary

A

abandonment a legal term for leaving an ill or injured person before an equal or more highly trained person can assume responsibility for care.

advance directive a legal document that outlines a person's wishes regarding his or her own health care.

airway adjunct a device designed to assist in keeping an open and clear airway.

altered mental status a change or decrease in mental abilities or responsiveness.

amniotic fluid the clear watery substance inside the amniotic sac.

amniotic sac the fluid-filled sac that surrounds the developing fetus.

amputation an injury that occurs when a body part or limb is forcibly cut or torn from the body.

angina chest pain caused by an inadequate supply of blood to the heart muscle.

angulation a deformity that occurs when a bone is broken and is bent out of its normal shape.

anterior the front of the body; e.g., the navel (belly button) is located on the anterior abdomen.

arteries blood vessels that transport oxygen-rich blood under high pressure to the organs and cells of the body.

auscultation taking a blood pressure reading by listening through a stethoscope.

B

bag-mask device a device used to provide rescue breaths for a person with inadequate respirations; it consists of a bag, one-way-valve, and facemask.

bandage a length of cloth or gauzelike material that is designed to hold a dressing in place over a wound.

battery a legal term for forcing care on someone who does not want it.

birth canal the interior of the vagina.

blood pressure the measurement of the pressure of blood against the inside of the walls of the arteries.

body mechanics refers to the proper use of the body to facilitate moving and lifting with the goal of maximizing effectiveness and minimizing personal injury.

body substance isolation (BSI) precautions precautions taken to minimize exposure to blood and other potentially infectious material, typically through the use of protective gloves and eyewear.

brain attack (stroke) a condition caused by interruption of blood flow to a portion of the brain.

breach of duty a legal term referring to the occasion when someone who has a duty to provide care fails to do so.

breech birth occurs when the baby is not properly positioned inside the uterus during labor and presents buttocks (or limb) first instead of headfirst.

C

capillaries the smallest of vessels that transport oxygenated blood.

capillary refill the return of blood into capillaries after it has been forced out by fingertip pressure; normal refill time is two seconds.

central nervous system a body system that is responsible for involuntary functions, such as heartbeat, respirations, and temperature regulation; it is composed of the brain and the spinal cord.

cervical spine the neck bones; it is composed of seven vertebrae.

cervix the opening of the uterus.

chair lift a technique for moving an ill or injured person down stairs or out of a building.

chief complaint the one thing that is causing the ill or injured person pain or discomfort and is the reason for which help was called.

closed fracture an injury in which the skin remains intact at the fracture site.

clothes drag an emergent move; a technique by which a single responder can move an ill or injured person who is on the ground.

coccyx the tailbone, or final segment of the spinal column.

confidentiality the obligation to not share information about an event or a person's condition with anyone except those who are directly involved in the incident or the person's care.

consent permission to provide care.

contractions the shortening of the uterine muscles, which occurs at intervals before and during childbirth.

convulsions uncontrolled muscle contractions of the body.

cranium the skull.

cravat a triangular bandage that is folded to a width of about three inches and used to tie a splint or dressing in place.

crepitus a crackling or grating feeling or sound most commonly associated with broken bones.

critical incident stress the stress that one experiences when faced with a significant event.

crowning the bulging that occurs at the opening of the vagina when the baby's head is pushing from the inside.

cyanosis bluish color of the lips and nail beds; a sign of poor perfusion.

D

diabetes a condition that results when the body is unable to produce an adequate supply of insulin or when the body can no longer utilize insulin well.

diastolic pressure the pressure remaining in the arteries when the heart is at rest or between contractions; measured in millimeters of mercury (mm Hg).

dislocation an injury that occurs when one or more bones that make up a joint become displaced.

distal further from the torso (in reference to a limb); e.g., the hand is distal to the elbow.

dressing an absorbent pad typically made of gauze or similar material.

duty of care the responsibility to others to act according to the law.

E

emergency medical responder an individual who arrives first on the scene of an incident and takes action to save lives.

emergency medical services (EMS) a formalized system of highly trained individuals and specialized resources designed to respond to, care for, and transport victims of sudden injury and illness.

emergent move a move that is necessary when there is an immediate threat to an ill or injured person's life.

epilepsy a condition affecting the brain and causing seizures.

ethics the study of the principles (rules) that define behavior as right, good, and proper.

evisceration an open wound to the abdomen that results in the exposure of the intestines.

exposure the condition of being subjected to a fluid or substance capable of transmitting an infectious agent in a manner that may have a harmful effect.

expressed consent a type of consent that occurs when a conscious person gives permission for care.

extremity lift a technique for moving an ill or injured person who is on the ground and must be lifted onto a chair or stretcher.

F

fallopian tube the pair of tubes along which ova (eggs) travel from the ovaries to the uterus.

fetus a medical term that refers to the unborn child.

frostbite a condition that occurs when the tissues of the skin become frozen.

G

general impression a quick assessment of the seriousness of the situation performed upon arrival at the scene.

generalized seizure a common type of seizure that results in a loss of consciousness and uncontrolled muscle contractions of the body.

Good Samaritan laws laws that exist in all 50 states that are designed to encourage "passersby" to stop and render care to an ill or injured person by limiting the exposure to civil liability.

H

heart attack a condition that occurs when blood flow to the heart muscle is interrupted enough to cause muscle damage.

heat exhaustion a condition marked by dizziness, nausea, and weakness and caused by overheating of the body.

heat stroke a condition that occurs when the normal cooling mechanisms of the body are unable to keep the body cool.

hemostatic dressing a dressing that contains clotting agents.

hypothermia a generalized cooling of the body's core temperature.

I

immediate life threat any condition that is immediately harmful to the ill or injured person, such as a blocked airway, inadequate breathing, or uncontrolled bleeding.

imminent birth a situation in which the birth of a baby is highly likely to occur immediately or within minutes.

implied consent a form of consent used for unconscious people or people under the legal age of consent.

incident command system (ICS) an organized approach to dealing with a multiple-casualty incident.

inferior toward the feet; e.g., the chin is inferior to the mouth.

L

labor the process a woman's body goes through to deliver a fetus.

lateral toward the side of the body; e.g., the thumb is on the lateral side of the hand.

ligaments tough, fiber-like tissues that connect two or more bones, typically at a joint.

log roll a technique for moving an ill or injured person from his back to his side, or from a facedown position to a face-up position.

lumbar spine the lower back, and largest movable portion of the spine; it is composed of five vertebrae.

M

mandated reporter a person who is legally obligated to report any suspicion of abuse or neglect.

manual stabilization restriction of movement by the use of the injured person's or responder's own hands; also called self-splinting.

mechanism of injury refers to the general cause of a person's injury.

medial toward the midline of the body; e.g., the pinky is located on the medial side of the hand.

medical direction the oversight given to EMS providers by a physician.

Medical Director the physician in charge of an EMS system.

mentally competent refers to people who are of sound mind and judgment and are able to make appropriate decisions about their own medical care.

midline the center of the body; e.g., the navel is located on the abdomen directly on the midline.

multiple-casualty incident (MCI) an incident with more than one ill or injured person; any incident that overwhelms the normal Emergency Responders or resources.

N

nasal cannula a device that delivers oxygen into the person's nostrils by way of two small plastic prongs.

national incident management system (NIMS) a nationally standardized system developed by the federal government for managing large-scale incidents that involve multiple agencies.

nature of illness refers to the general cause of the ill person's complaint, such as difficulty breathing, chest pain, or dizziness.

negligence failure to exercise the care toward others that a reasonable or prudent person would in the circumstances.

nonrebreather mask a device consisting of a facemask with a one-way valve and a reservoir bag; used to deliver high concentrations of oxygen.

O

occlusive dressing a dressing that does not allow air to pass through.

open fracture an injury in which the soft tissue of the skin has been broken at or near the fracture site.

ovary the organ that produces the egg, or ovum.

overdose occurs when a person ingests too much of a substance such as a medication.

P

palpation using the hands to assess the body.

paralysis the loss of mobility to an area of the body.

pathogens germs that can cause disease.

peripheral nervous system a body system that connects the CNS to the limbs and organs by way of nerves; it is composed of all the nerves and nerve endings that extend from the spinal cord throughout the body.

personal protective equipment equipment, such as protective gloves and eyewear, that minimizes exposure to pathogens.

placenta a complex vascular organ that permits the exchange of blood and other nutrients necessary to keep the fetus alive and growing.

placenta previa occurs when the placenta implants itself or grows over the opening of the cervix.

position of function the natural relaxed position of a body part, specifically the hand or foot.

postictal an unresponsive state of the body that follows a generalized seizure.

posterior the back of the body; e.g., the shoulder blades are located on the posterior side of the torso.

precipitous birth a very fast labor and delivery.

pressure regulator a device used to reduce the pressure of a gas (oxygen) so that it can be easily controlled and delivered to an ill or injured person.

primary assessment the first step in the actual assessment of the ill or injured person; an examination that includes mental status, airway, breathing, circulation, and bleeding.

prolapsed cord occurs when the umbilical cord presents through the vagina before the baby's head crowns.

prone lying facedown.

protocols emergency care guidelines developed in cooperation with the Medical Director; they provide EMS personnel and some Emergency Responders with recommended procedures for emergency care.

proximal closer to the torso (in reference to a limb); e.g., the shoulder is proximal to the elbow.

R

reassessment a recheck of the ABCs, chief complaint, vital signs, and interventions.

recovery position lying on the left side; a position that engages gravity to help keep the ill or injured person's airway clear.

respiration one inspiration plus one exhalation of breath; also the exchange of oxgyen and carbon dioxide at the cellular level.

respiratory arrest the complete stoppage of any attempts to breathe.

respiratory difficulty an increased work of breathing and an increased breathing rate; also called shortness of breath.

S

sacrum a triangular segment at the base of the spine; the upper part connects with the last lumbar vertebra and the bottom part with the coccyx; it is composed of five fused bones.

scene size-up an overview of the scene to identify any immediate or potential hazards at the scene of the emergency as well as the need for additional resources.

secondary assessment a thorough examination of the ill or injured person, beginning with the chief complaint and including evaluation of vital signs.

shock a condition that results when the organs and cells of the body do not receive an adequate supply of well-oxygenated blood.

sign something that can be seen or measured, such as bleeding, swelling, bruising, or how fast or slow an ill or injured person is breathing.

sling a triangular cloth device used to immobilize an injured arm.

sphygmomanometer a device used to measure blood pressure.

splint a device used to immobilize an injured extremity.

sprain an injury that occurs when two or more bones that make up a joint are stretched beyond their capacity.

stair chair a device specifically designed to allow responders to move an ill or injured person down stairs safely.

standard precautions the set of infection-prevention practices health-care personnel use when caring for ill and injured people.

START triage system a structured approach to triaging multiple injured individuals based on specific criteria.

stethoscope an instrument used for listening to sounds within the body.

strain an injury that occurs when a muscle is stretched or "pulled" beyond its capacity.

stress tension, or a state of mental or emotional strain or suspense; the normal response to an abnormal situation or incident.

stressor any event or situation that places extraordinary demands on a person's mental and/or emotional resources.

suction catheter a device used to suction fluids from a person's mouth and/or nose.

superior toward the head; e.g., the nose is superior to the mouth.

supine lying face up.

swathe a large cravat usually made of cloth, used to secure a sling or splint to the body.

symptom something that cannot be seen but that the ill or injured person feels and can describe, such as pain, nausea, or dizziness.

systolic pressure the pressure inside the arteries when the heart is contracting; measured in millimeters of mercury (mm Hg).

T

tendons the structures at the end of each muscle that attach directly to the bone.

thoracic spine the middle segment of the spine; these bones articulate with the ribs; it is composed of 12 vertebrae.

tourniquet a device that when applied to a limb stops all blood flow past the device.

trimester a period of three months; commonly used to describe the progression of a pregnancy.

tripod position a position in which a person who is having difficulty breathing will get into so it is easier to breathe; position in which hands are on the knees and shoulders held high.

U

umbilical cord the structure that connects the fetus to the placenta.

uterus the muscular organ that houses the developing fetus.

V

veins vessels that transport blood depleted of oxygen under low pressure from the organs and cells and return it to the heart.

ventilations rescue breaths.

vital signs the key signs of life, which include respirations, pulse, skin signs, and blood pressure.

Index

D

Deceased, triage evaluation, 167
Decision-making process, 14
Decontamination, 214
Deep femoral artery, 41
Deformities
    musculoskeletal injury, 140
    in physical examination, 85
Delayed, triage evaluation, 167
Delivery. *See also* Childbirth
    ABC monitoring, 180
    assisting with, 178–180
    body substance isolation (BSI) precautions, 178
    imminent, signs and symptoms, 176–177
    mother care, 181
    newborn care, 180
    normal, 178–180
    OB kit and, 177
    placenta, 180
    preparing for, 177
Dental injuries, 129–130
Dermis, 45
Diabetes. *See also* Illnesses
    defined, 102
    management, 102–103
    priorities of care, 103
    signs and symptoms, 103
Diaphragm, 38
Diastolic pressure, 186
Directional anatomical terms, 37
Dislocations, 138
Distal, 37, 38
Distal extremity assessment. *See also* Musculoskeletal injuries
    capillary refill, 141, 142
    characteristics, 141
    illustrated, 141
    movement, 142
    sensation, 142
Do not resuscitate (DNR) orders. *See also* Advance directives
    defined, 19–20
    differences in, 20
    illustrated, 20
    initiation, 19–20
    understanding, 20–21
    validity, 20
Documentation. *See also* Assessment
    elements, 92
    forms, 92
    importance, 92
    pulse, 89

Dorsal pedis artery, 41
Dressings
    defined, 120
    hemostatic, 121, 122
    occlusive, 121
Duty, 16

E

EAPs. *See* Emergency action plans
Elbow, 42, 137
Elderly, abuse and neglect, 19
Emergencies
    cold-related, 107–108
    heat-related, 108–110
    illness-related, 97–99
    on-site, managing, 6–7
    recognition, 5
Emergency action plans (EAPs)
    activating, 9
    defined, 8
    safety and emergency procedures, 26
    understanding, 10
Emergency care. *See* Care
Emergency Medical Responder (EMR), 4
Emergency medical service (EMS) personnel
    levels of training, 4
    responders arriving before, 3
Emergency medical services (EMS) system
    accessing, 8–10
    activating, 7
    components, 3
    defined, 3
    levels of care, 4
    levels of training in, 5
    Medical Director in charge of, 8
    radio activation of, 8
    state-to-state differences, 5
Emergency Medical Technician (EMT), 4
Emergency oxygen, 193–203
Emergency Responder
    as advocate for the ill and injured, 7
    care expectation, 5
    as care providers, 5
    compassion, 14
    defined, 2
    ethics, 13
    interaction with Medical Director, 8
    liability, 15
    lifelong learning, 7–8
    in multiple-casualty incidents, 165–166
    role of, 6–8
    as safety advocate, 6–7
    stresses, 29–32

M

Mandated reporters, 19
Mandible, 42, 62
Manual stabilization
head and neck, 158–159
musculoskeletal injury, 143
spine injury, 158–159
Masks
bag, 72, 200–203
defined, 29
nonrebreather, 200–201
in rescue breathing, 71
Maxilla, 42
MCIs. *See* Multiple-casualty incidents
Mechanism of injury
defined, 78
in scene size-up, 80
spine injury, 155–157
Medial, 37
Medical direction, 8
Medical Director, 8
Medical emergencies. *See* Emergencies
Medical history, 83
Medications, in history, 83
Mental status
defined, 81
in primary assessment, 81–82
scale, 82
START triage system, 169
Mentally competent, 17
Metacarpals (hand), 42, 137
Metatarsals (foot), 42, 137
Midline, 37
Minor, triage evaluation, 167
Minors. *See also* Children
implied consent and, 17
refusal of care and, 18
Mother, childbirth
care of, 181
evaluation, 175–176
privacy, 178
Mouth-to-barrier-device ventilation, 71
Mouth-to-mask ventilation, 71
Moves. *See also* Body mechanics; Lifts
body mechanics and, 51–52
clothes drag, 57
common, 52–57
communication and, 52
decision, 49–50
emergent, 50–51
improper, 51
log roll, 54–55
nonemergent, 50–51
number of people for, 51

recovery position, 53–54
star chair, 56
Multiple-casualty incidents (MCIs)
defined, 165
Emergency Responder's role, 165–166
incident command system (ICS) and, 166
national incident management system (NIMS) and, 166
scene safety, 165
triage, 167–170
Muscles
functions, 43, 136
illustrated and labeled, 43
Musculoskeletal injuries, 138–148
angulation, 140
care priority, 140
caring for, 142–143
children and, 143
closed, 138
deformities, 140
determining, 139
dislocation, 138
distal extremity assessment, 141–142
fracture, 138
immobilizing, 143–148
manual stabilization, 143
open, 138
signs and symptoms, 139
sprain, 138
strain, 138
types of, 138
Musculoskeletal system, 136–137
elements, 42
muscles illustration, 43
skeleton illustration, 42, 137

N

Nasal cannula. *See also* Oxygen delivery; Oxygen therapy
application, 198–200
application illustration, 199
defined, 198
Nasal cavity, 62
Nasal passage, 39
National incident management system (NIMS), 166
Natural disasters, 24
Nature of illness
defined, 77–78
in scene size-up, 80
Neck
injury, in scene size-up, 80
manual stabilization, 158–159
physical exam, 85, 87
in skeletal system, 42, 137

steps for providing, 73
vomiting and, 71
Respiration assessment. *See also* Assessment
  depth, 90
  difficulty, 91
  illustrated, 90
  process, 90–91
  rate, 90
Respirations, START triage system, 168
Respiratory arrest, 69
Respiratory difficulty. *See also* Breathing
  caring for, 70
  common causes, 68–69
  defined, 68
  respiratory arrest versus, 69
  signs and symptoms, 69
Respiratory system
  elements, 39
  function of, 39–40
  illustrated, 39
Responding, reckless, 25
Responsive person
  complete airway obstruction, 63–64
  partial airway obstruction, 62, 64
Ribs, 42, 137
Rickettsia, biological agent, 210
Riot-control agents, 213
Risks
  airway management, 64
  emergency scene, 24
  helping others and, 25
  improper body mechanics, 51
  minimizing, 25–26
  unreasonable, 25

S

Sacrum
  defined, 155
  illustrated, 42, 155
Safety
  body substance isolation (BSI), 27–29
  childbirth, 176
  cleanup, 29
  emergency scene risks and, 24
  importance of, 24–29
  minimizing risk and, 25–26
  multiple-casualty incidents, 165
  oxygen cylinder, 195
  pathogens, 26–27
  precautions, 27–29
  pressure regulators, 197
  scene, 7
  in scene size-up, 80

self, 7
  as top priority, 25
Safety advocates
  care as, 7
  champion as, 6
  Emergency Responders as, 6–7
Scapula (shoulder blade), 42, 137
Scene size-up. *See also* Assessment
  additional resources, 80
  defined, 79
  ill persons, 98
  nature of illness/mechanism of injury, 80
  number of ill/injured persons, 80
  possible neck/back injuries, 80
  safety, 80
Second stage, labor, 175
Secondary assessment, 83–87. *See also* Assessment
  chief complaint and, 84
  components, 83
  defined, 83
  history, 83–84
  ill person, 99
  physical examination, 84–87
Seizures. *See also* Illnesses
  cause, 100
  defined, 100
  generalized, 100
  postictal state, 101
  priorities of care, 100–101
  signs and symptoms, 100
SETUP (stop, environment, traffic, unknown hazard, protect), 26
Severe allergic reaction. *See also* Illnesses
  autoinjector use illustration, 113
  defined, 112
  priorities of care, 113
  signs and symptoms, 112–113
Sharing information, 15
Shock, 119
Signs. *See also* Symptoms
  altered mental status, 100
  bites and stings, 111
  brain attack, 101–102
  breathing problems, 105
  chest pain, 104
  cold-related emergencies, 107–108
  cyanogens, 212
  defined, 79
  diabetes, 103
  examples, 79
  head injury, 153
  heat-related emergencies, 109
  in history, 83

Symptoms. *See also* Signs
  altered mental status, 100
  bites and stings, 111
  brain attack, 101–102
  breathing problems, 105
  chest pain, 104
  cold-related emergencies, 107–108
  cyanogens, 212
  defined, 79
  diabetes, 103
  examples, 79
  head injury, 153
  heat-related emergencies, 109
  in history, 83
  illness, 97–98
  imminent birth, 176–177
  internal bleeding, 125
  musculoskeletal injury, 139–140
  nerve agents, 211
  protection in treating, 154
  pulmonary agents, 212
  riot-control agents, 213
  seizures, 100
  severe allergic reaction, 112–113
  shock, 119
  spine injury, 157
  vesicant agents, 212
Systolic pressure, 186

T

Tarsals (ankle), 42, 137
Temporal bone, 42
Tendons, 137
Terrorism
  biological agents, 209
  chemical agents, 210–213
  decontamination and, 214
  defined, 208
  effects of, 209
  Emergency Responder role, 213
  nuclear/radiological agents, 209–210
Third stage, labor, 175
Thoracic spine
  defined, 154
  illustrated, 137, 155
Thyroid cartilage (Adam's apple),
    39, 62
Thyroid gland, 62
Tibia, 42, 137
Tongue
  in head-tilt/chin-lift maneuver, 65
  in upper airway anatomy, 62

Tonsils, 62
Tourniquets
  after application of, 123
  application of, 123
  application using a cravat, 124
  for bleeding control, 123
  commercial, application of, 125
  defined, 123
  use of, 123
Toxins, biological agent, 210
Trachea, 39, 40, 62
Traffic, before entering emergency scene, 26
Training
  Advanced Emergency Medical Technician
      (AEMT), 4
  continuing, 13
  Emergency Medical Responder (EMR), 4
  Emergency Medical Technician (EMT), 4
  gap, 5–6
  Paramedic, 4
  standardized course, 6
  state-to-state differences, 5
Triage, 167–170
  components, 167–168
  deceased, 167
  defined, 167
  delayed, 167
  immediate, 167
  minor, 167
  START system, 168–170
  tags, 169
  walking wounded assistance, 169
Triceps, 43
Trimesters, 174
Tripod position, 105–106

U

Ulna, 42, 137
Umbilical cord, 174
Unknown hazard, before entering emergency scene,
    26
Unresponsive person airway management,
    65–68.
    See also Airway management
  assessing, 64–66
  clearing, 66–68
  head-tilt/chin-lift maneuver, 65
  jaw-thrust maneuver, 65–66
  oropharyngeal airways (OPAs) and,
    203
Unresponsive persons, spinal injury care, 158
Ureter, 38
Uterus, 174